ANTIBIOTIC RESISTANCE: ORIGINS, EVOLUTION, SELECTION AND SPREAD

The Ciba Foundation is an international scientific and educational charity (Registered Charity No. 313574). It was established in 1947 by the Swiss chemical and pharmaceutical company of CIBA Limited—now Ciba-Geigy Limited. The Foundation operates independently in London under English trust law.

The Ciba Foundation exists to promote international cooperation in biological, medical and chemical research. It organizes about eight international multidisciplinary symposia each year on topics that seem ready for discussion by a small group of research workers. The papers and discussions are published in the Ciba Foundation symposium series. The Foundation also holds many shorter meetings (not published), organized by the Foundation itself or by outside scientific organizations. The staff always welcome suggestions for future meetings.

The Foundation's house at 41 Portland Place, London W1N 4BN, provides facilities for meetings of all kinds. Its Media Resource Service supplies information to journalists on all scientific and technological topics. The library, open five days a week to any graduate in science or medicine, also provides information on scientific meetings throughout the world and answers general enquiries on biomedical and chemical subjects. Scientists from any part of the world may stay in the house during working visits to London.

Ciba Foundation Symposium 207

ANTIBIOTIC RESISTANCE: ORIGINS, EVOLUTION, SELECTION AND SPREAD

1997

JOHN WILEY & SONS

Chichester · New York · Weinheim · Brisbane · Singapore · Toronto

Copyright © Ciba Foundation 1997
Published in 1997 by John Wiley & Sons Ltd,
Baffins Lane, Chichester,
West Sussex PO19 1UD, England

National 01243 779777
International (+44) 1243 779777
e-mail (for orders and customer service enquiries): cs-books@wiley.co.uk
Visit our Home Page on http://www.wiley.co.uk
or http://www.wiley.com

Other Wiley Editorial Offices

John Wiley & Sons, Inc., 605 Third Avenue,
New York, NY 10158-0012, USA

VCH Verlagsgesellschaft mbH, Pappelallee 3,
D-69469 Weinheim, Germany

Jacaranda Wiley Ltd, 33 Park Road, Milton,
Queensland 4064, Australia

John Wiley & Sons (Canada) Ltd, 22 Worcester Road,
Rexdale, Ontario M9W 1L1, Canada

John Wiley & Sons (Asia) Pte Ltd, 2 Clementi Loop #02-01,
Jin Xing Distripark, Singapore 0512

Ciba Foundation Symposium 207
ix+250 pages, 26 figures, 32 tables

Library of Congress Cataloging-in-Publication Data

Antibiotic resistance : origins, evolution, selection, and spread.
        p.   cm. — (Ciba Foundation symposium ; 207)
    "Editors: Derek J. Chadwick (organizer) and Jamie Goode" — Contents
p.
    Includes bibliographical references and index.
    ISBN 0-471-97105-7 (alk. paper)
    1. Drug resistance in microorganisms–Congresses.   I. Chadwick,
Derek.   II. Goode, Jamie.   III. Series
    [DNLM: 1. Antibiotics — pharmacology — congresses.   2. Drug
Resistance, Microbial — congresses.   W3 C161F v.207 1997 / QV 350
A6267 1997]
    QR177.A566   1997
    616′ .01 — dc21
    DNLM/DLC
    for Library of Congress   96-29697
                                                                  CIP

British Library Cataloguing in Publication Data

A catalogue record for this book is available from the British Library

ISBN 0 471 97105 7

Typeset in 10/12pt Garamond by Dobbie Typesetting Limited, Tavistock, Devon.
Printed and bound in Great Britain by Biddles Ltd, Guildford.
This book is printed on acid-free paper responsibly manufactured from sustainable forestation,
for which at least two trees are planted for each one used for paper production.

Contents

Participants

F. Baquero   Department of Microbiology, Ramón y Cajal Hospital, National Institute of Health (INSALUD), 28034 Madrid, Spain

M. L. Bennish   Division of Geographic Medicine and Infectious Disease, Departments of Medicine and Pediatrics, New England Medical Center, Tufts University School of Medicine, 750 Washington Street, Box 041, Boston, MA 02111, USA

K. Bush   Department of Microbial Biochemistry, Astra Research Center Boston, 128 Sidney Street, Cambridge, MA 02139, USA

M. L. Cohen   Division of Bacterial and Mycotic Diseases, National Center for Infectious Disease, Centers for Disease Control and Prevention, 1600 Clifton Road, C09, Atlanta, GA 30333, USA

J. V. Copeland   SmithKline Beecham Consumer Healthcare, Three New Horizons Court, Brentford, Middlesex, UK

J. E. Davies   Department of Microbiology and Immunology, University of British Columbia, #300–6174 University Boulevard, Vancouver, BC, Canada V6T 1Z3

R. Gaynes   Hospital Infections Program, MS E-55, Centers for Disease Control and Prevention, 1600 Clifton Road, Altanta, GA 30333, USA

H. Giamarellou   Infectious Diseases Section, Athens University School of Medicine, 1st Department of Propedeutic Medicine, Laiko, General Hospital, GR 115 27, Athens, Greece

R. M. Hall   CSIRO, Division of Biomolecular Engineering, Sydney Laboratory, PO Box 184, North Ryde, NSW 2113, Australia

P. Huovinen   Antimicrobial Research Laboratory, National Public Health Institute, PO Box 57, SF-20521 Turku, Finland

R. E. Lenski   Center for Microbial Ecology, Michigan State University, East Lansing, MI 48824, USA

S. A. Lerner   Division of Infectious Diseases, Wayne State University, School of Medicine, 4160 John R, Suite 2140, Detroit, MI 48201, USA

B. R. Levin   Department of Biology, Emory University, 1510 Clifton Road, Atlanta, GA 30322, USA

S. B. Levy *(Chairman)*   Center for Adaptation Genetics and Drug Resistance and the Departments of Molecular Biology and Microbiology and of Medicine, Tufts University School of Medicine, 136 Harrison Avenue, Boston, MA 02111, USA

M. Lipsitch *(Ciba Foundation Bursar)*   Department of Biology, Emory University, 1510 Clifton Road, Atlanta, GA 30322, USA

G. Miller   Schering-Plough Research Institute, 2015 Galloping Hill Road, Kenilworth, NJ 07033–0539, USA

W. C. Noble   Department of Microbial Diseases, Institute of Dermatology, UMDS, St Thomas' Hospital, Lambeth Palace Road, London SE1 7EH, UK

M. Nowak   Department of Zoology, University of Oxford, South Parks Road, Oxford OX1 3PS, UK

L. J. V. Piddock   Department of Infection, The Medical School, University of Birmingham, Egbaston, Birmingham B15 2TT, UK

M. C. Roberts Department of Pathobiology, Box 357238, School of Public Health and Community Medicine, University of Washington, Seattle, WA 98195–7238, USA

O. Sköld   Division of Microbiology, Department of Pharmaceutical Biosciences, Uppsala University, PO Box 581, S-751 23 Uppsala, Sweden

R. A. Skurray   School of Biological Sciences, Macleay Building A12, University of Sydney, NSW 2006, Australia

B. G. Spratt   School of Biological Sciences, University of Sussex, Falmer, Brighton BN1 9QG, UK

A. O. Summers   University of Georgia, Department of Microbiology, Athens, GA 30602, USA

E. J. Threlfall   Laboratory of Enteric Pathogens, PHLS Central Public Health Laboratory, 61 Colindale Avenue, London NW9 5HT, UK

W. Witte   Robert Koch-Institut, Wernigerode Branch, Burgstraße 37, D-38855 Wernigerode, Germany

Antibiotic resistance: an ecological imbalance

Stuart B. Levy

Center for Adaptation Genetics and Drug Resistance and the Departments of Molecular Biology and Microbiology and of Medicine, Tufts University School of Medicine, 136 Harrison Avenue, Boston, MA 02111, USA

Abstract. Antibiotic resistance thwarts the treatment of infectious diseases worldwide. Although a number of factors can be identified which contribute to the problem, clearly the *antibiotic* as a selective agent and the *resistance gene* as the vehicle of resistance are the two most important, making up a 'drug resistance equation'. Both are needed in order for a clinical problem to arise. Given sufficient time and quantity of antibiotic, drug resistance will eventually appear. But a public health problem is not inevitable if the two components of the drug resistance equation are kept in check. Enhancing the emergence of resistance is the ease by which resistance determinants and resistant bacteria can spread locally and globally, selected by widespread use of the same antibiotics in people, animal husbandry and agriculture. Antibiotics are societal drugs. Each individual use contributes to the sum total of society's antibiotic exposure. In a broader sense, the resistance problem is ecological. In the framework of natural competition between susceptible and resistant bacteria, antibiotic use has encouraged growth of the resistant strains, leading to an imbalance in prior relationships between susceptible and resistant bacteria. To restore efficacy to earlier antibiotics and to maintain the success of new antibiotics that are introduced, we need to use antibiotics in a way which assures an ecological balance that favours the predominance of susceptible bacterial flora.

1997 Antibiotic resistance: origins, evolution, selection and spread. Wiley, Chichester (Ciba Foundation Symposium 207) p 1–14

In large part, bacteria live in harmony with other inhabitants of the earth. Although some infections are caused by bacteria for which humans are a specific host, in most instances the infections follow entry of bacteria into the body by chance. Over the past 50 years, the classic treatment of bacterial infectious diseases has been antibiotics, the discovery of which vastly changed the relationship between bacteria and people. Today we are witnessing another change, that is, among the bacteria themselves.

While diversity characterizes the microbial flora, antibiotic use has led to a further subgrouping into those bacteria that are susceptible and those that are resistant to antibiotics. Prior to antibiotic introduction, the large majority of commensal and infectious bacteria associated with people were susceptible to these agents. Over the ensuing five decades the mounting increase in the use of antibiotics, not only in people, but also in animals and in agriculture, has delivered a selection unprecedented in the history of evolution (Levy 1992). The powerful killing and growth inhibitory effects of antibiotics have reduced the numbers of susceptible strains, leading to the propagation of resistant variants. These have eventually evolved into prominent members of the microbial flora. The antibiotic susceptibility profile of bacteria on the skin of people today, and in the environments of hospitals and homes, is very different from what it was in the pre-antibiotic era, and even 10 years ago. Multidrug resistance is commonly found in bacteria which cause infections as well as in commensal organisms which colonize our intestinal tract, skin and upper respiratory tracts. The resistant bacteria are the survivors of the antibiotic selection which has been taking place within various segments of society.

Microbes circulate everywhere, and there is a continual exchange among the different human, animal and agricultural hosts. We do not know which bacteria are resistant and which are susceptible. As has been suggested, it would be very helpful if we had a system by which we could see resistant bacteria in different colours, distinguishing them from susceptible bacterial populations (O'Brien & Stelling 1995). We could then determine the environments needing remediation, i.e. a return of susceptible flora.

Antibiotics are unique therapeutics. They treat more than just the individual. They treat the environment and in that way they affect society. This characteristic of antibiotics is why today's society is facing one of its gravest public health problems — numerous infectious bacteria with resistance to many, and in some cases to all, available antibiotics. Antibiotic resistance exemplifies *par excellence* Darwinism: surviving strains have emerged under the protection and selection by the antibiotic. Use of the same antibiotics in all parts of the world has led to the emergence of resistant bacteria that find ready havens for propagation wherever they move.

Antibiotics have also revealed the genetic fluidity of bacteria in terms of their ability to exchange genetic traits among genera and species which are evolutionarily millennia apart. Antibiotic resistance genes on plasmids and transposons flow to and from Gram-positive and Gram-negative bacteria, and among bacteria which inhabit vastly different ecological niches.

In assessing the antibiotic resistance problem, we can identify a number of factors which have contributed and continue to impact on the emergence of resistance. The leading two are the antibiotic itself and the resistance determinant. They make up what I have called the 'drug resistance equation.' (Fig. 1) (Levy 1994) The two entities ebb and flow to affect the magnitude of the clinical drug resistance problem. If either is

---

Antibiotic + Resistance trait → Antibiotic resistance problem

FIG. 1.   The drug resistance equation.

absent, a drug resistance problem will not emerge; but given the presence of both the antibiotic and a resistance trait, drug resistant bacteria will be selected and propagated. To these two factors, we can add spread of resistant bacteria themselves and the cell to cell spread of the resistance traits. It is no wonder that an environment can become rapidly populated with different kinds of resistant bacteria.

Antibiotics and the emergence of resistance: the selection density

Antibiotics were initially developed for the treatment of infectious diseases in people. Their miraculous effects led to their being solicited and used for the treatment of animals and eventually plants. The same ones are being used in all three areas. Thus, an enormous worldwide selective pressure has occurred. Antibiotics are used both internally and externally to control bacterial problems for society, maintaining the health of people, animals and agricultural crops. If different antibiotics had been chosen for animals and agriculture than those used in people, we might be witnessing a lower level of resistance today. But, in fact, with each ensuing year, 4–5% more antibiotics have been produced, developed and used. In the USA alone, an estimated 160 million prescriptions for antibiotics were written last year and over 50 million pounds were produced for use in people, animals and agriculture.

There are two major effects of an antibiotic: therapeutically, it treats the invading infectious organism, but it also eliminates other, or non-disease producing, bacteria in its wake. The latter do, in fact, contribute to the diversity of the ecosystem and the natural balance between susceptible and resistant strains. The consequence of antibiotic use is, therefore, the disruption of the natural microbial ecology. This alteration may be revealed in the emergence of types of bacteria which are very different from those previously found there, or drug resistant variants of the same ones that were already present. The dominance acquired by these new strains in the treated environment is directly linked to the intrinsic or acquired resistance to the antibiotics being used.

To a large extent, the reversibility of the selection process is dependent on repopulation by the original susceptible bacteria. Their residual numbers will be related to the total amount of selective drug used in that environment. This relationship suggests that it is the density of the antibiotic, i.e. the total quantity applied, the number of individuals (people, animals, plants) treated, and the size of the geographic area affected, which quantitatively and qualitatively affects microbial ecology. This concept translates directly into a 'density' selection process which affects that ecology (Fig. 2). The introduction of an antibiotic into an environment has the eventual effect of killing-off most, if not all, of the resident susceptible strains. Any resistant survivors will then have a chance to propagate and take over. But adjacent to that selective environment, and encroaching on it, are untreated, susceptible strains which are still potential competitors for the treated area, if given the opportunity. The size of the area selected for resistance will be related to the total amount of antibiotic used and the geographical extent of its influence. It further relies on the potential for susceptible strains to return after the selective event. One would not expect the same ecological

Amount of Antibiotic	*per*	Individual	*per*	Geographic Area

FIG. 2.   Selection density.

effect if a hundred pounds of antibiotic were distributed among 20 animals as compared to 20 000 animals. As long as the dosage of antibiotic is above its growth-inhibitory concentration, a greater effect will be seen in the larger numbers of animals being treated — as they will be propagating a thousand times more resistant bacteria. Likewise, the ecological effect of two individuals treated in one room will be different from two being treated in two different rooms or homes. The selection of antibiotic resistance is, therefore, greatly affected by the numbers being treated as well as the size of the treatment area and the numbers of susceptible bacteria surviving the treatment.

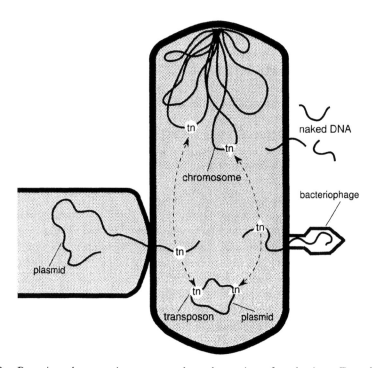

FIG. 3.   Bacteria exchange resistance genes through a variety of mechanisms. Extrachromosomal plasmids can deliver genes they bear from one bacterium to other bacteria of different types. Small DNA elements, called transposons (tn), can move among various DNAs: plasmids, chromosomes and bacteriophages. DNA can enter the cell on plasmids through cell to cell contact (conjugation) between two cells, by bacteriophage introduction, or by cellular uptake of naked DNA. (Adapted from Fig. 4.3 in Levy 1992.)

Genetics of drug resistance and spread

The emergence of resistant bacteria raises concern about the bacteria and their progeny and also the extent that they can spread to other environments. The bacterium itself is the focus, if the resistance trait is linked solely to that bacterium and cannot be shared by others. This is, however, not the case with most resistance traits in the majority of bacteria. They have evolved extrachromosomal replicating genes called plasmids and their associated transposons which allow rapid and very broad dissemination of genes (Fig. 3). Gene transfer crosses species and genus barriers (DeFlaun & Levy 1989). Thus, resistant enterococci selected in one environment can pass resistance genes not only to other members of their own genus and species but also to other organisms in other genera. Staphylococci share their plasmids with *Listeria; Escherichia coli* can share genes with other members of the *Enterobacteriaceae* as well as the pseudomonads and *Neisseria*, just to mention a few. In fact, the same tetracycline resistance determinants can be found among Gram-positive and Gram-negative bacteria as well as in the mycobacterium (Roberts 1997, this volume). The genetic flexibility and versatility of bacteria have therefore contributed largely to the efficiency by which antibiotic resistance has spread among bacteria and among environments globally. However, it is equally evident that the transfer event has no consequence unless the antibiotic selection is there. Thus, the emergence and maintenance of bacterial resistance relies on the interrelationship between the resistance determinant and the antibiotic.

Reversal of resistance

Data on the reversal of the resistance selection offer further insights into the selection process. The faecal flora of a volunteer, myself, taking tetracycline for five days was examined. Initially tetracycline resistance was present at a low level; it peaked within two days of tetracycline use. After five days, tetracycline was stopped, but the resistance frequency declined very slowly. The rate of loss did not mimic the rate of gain of resistance: it took 15 days to return to the initial pre-antibiotic level (Levy 1986). Antibiotics are so powerful that they provide rapid selection for a new resistant breed, but when you remove the antibiotic, a reversal is slow in coming. The resistant bacteria selected by tetracycline are no less 'fit' than the susceptible flora; hence they continue to propagate and persist.

We did similar studies among chickens excreting *E. coli* with multi-resistance plasmids. They did not lose the *E. coli*, despite multiple cleanings of the cage over several months (Levy 1986). However, this was a closed environment, and there was no easy route of entry for susceptible strains. Moreover, the resistant bacteria were clearly not disadvantaged by bearing resistance. When the cages were relocated to different sites around the barn, the surrounding environment was altered and the chickens' flora slowly returned to a more susceptible one (Levy 1986). In another study, we added four chickens excreting a resistant flora to 10 other chickens excreting a susceptible flora. Resistance was lost; the susceptible flora won out. For an immediate change in resistance frequency, the result relies on numbers, not large differences in bacterial fitness. Moreover, there is no active counter-selective force which propels repopulation with susceptible strains.

In the short term, the resistant bacteria were not less fit than the susceptible ones, so we did not observe a rapid shift from resistance to susceptibility. However, in the long term such changes have been documented in hospitals (Giamarellou & Antoniadou 1997, this volume) and on farms (Levy et al 1976) when antibiotics have been removed. But it takes time. In some instances, a newly gained plasmid is not stably kept in its new host. Early on, this instability will help in reversing the resistance. However, with time, the plasmid and bacteria may develop a synergistic relationship whereby both are needed for growth, demonstrating a phenomenon to be discussed later in this symposium (Lenski 1997, this volume). Still, the evidence suggests that, given a 'ready and willing' susceptible flora, a resistance predominance can be overturned if antibiotics are removed.

The resistance reservoir

Resistance genes reside not only in disease-causing organisms, but in commensal organisms as well. These normally harmless bacteria, such as *E. coli* or enterococcus, can cause a fatal illness if the person is immunocompromised. Moreover, these bacteria harbour resistance genes which can spread to the bacterial strains that do cause infection. Unfortunately, these reservoirs are not being examined very much.

People today harbour many multidrug resistant bacteria. In a study of faecal flora from an ambulatory community, we found that 40% of people on antibiotics carried two or more resistances in 10% of their *E. coli*; 25% had three or more resistances, and 10% had four or more (Levy et al 1988). People excrete resistant *E. coli* at the 50% level, even when not consuming antibiotics (Levy et al 1988). High carriage levels of resistant faecal flora have been reported from Holland (Bonten et al 1992), and elsewhere (Calva et al 1992, Leistevuo et al 1996). Resistant bacteria are plentiful in the environment, providing evidence for an environment in a state of imbalance. While not necessarily inflicting harm, they certainly reflect a significant selection process.

One source of resistant bacteria is food. A large number of drug resistant Gram-negative bacteria are asssociated with uncooked foods (Levy 1984). In the great majority of instances these bacteria pose no health problem. But they too tell us a lot about the environmental imbalance. A study from France assessed the contribution of food bacteria to the intestinal flora by examining the same volunteers when eating normal or sterilized food (Corpet 1988). Tetracycline resistance in the faecal flora was high when the volunteers were eating normal, non-sterilized food for 21 days, but dropped dramatically when the diet was shifted to sterilized food for 17 days (Table 1).

Besides selecting resistant variants, antibiotics can affect the ecology by changing the types of organisms there. New opportunistic infectious disease agents, intrinsically resistant to the antibiotic in use, can emerge and predominate. For instance, the use of second and third generation cephalosporins in hospitals, introduced for Gram-negative bacteria, selected the normally harmless enterococcus, which is intrinsically resistant to these antibiotics. The enterococci, selected by these drugs, have now become prominent members of the

TABLE 1 Log number of total and tetracycline-resistant lactose-fermenting enteric bacilli from six volunteers on a sterile diet

Control diet (21 d)		Sterile diet (17 d)	
Total	Tet^R	Total	Tet^R
7.4 ± 0.7	5.2 ± 1.3	6.9 ± 1.0	2.5 ± 1.4

Data for the control and sterile diets are means ± SD for 21 and 17 daily counts, respectively. Tet^R denotes tetracycline resistant. Data from Corpet (1988).

hospital acquired flora. Moreover, the organism has emerged with its own multiplicity of resistances, e.g. to aminoglycosides and vancomycin. It is a likely potential donor of vancomycin resistance to the staphylococcus. Replacement of an endogenous flora with a new flora as a consequence of antibiotic use is an important concept that is too often disregarded. It has a significant impact to our health.

If one is thinking about using an antibiotic to target the disease-causing organism, which, of course, is the magic of these drugs, one has to think about the other bacteria as well. If the antibiotic's sphere of influence is large, then its ecological effect will be large. As we widen antibiotic usage from the individual to the hospitals and the community, we see more and more effect on the susceptible strains. Some have talked about spraying hospital rooms with susceptible commensal organisms to replace and compete with the disease agents. It is an approach worth considering.

Overall, let's focus not just on the antibiotic, but also on the susceptible flora. Susceptible bacteria should be our teammates in confronting and reversing the resistance problem.

Why all the current publicity?

Why has so much recent attention been given to a field that some of us in this room have been working in for decades? Many journalists writing about it are directed by a personal experience. Many of these writers, or their editors, have children who have, or have had, ear infections or other infections that did not respond to antibiotics. The pneumococcus, whether the real culprit or not, has clearly brought the drug resistance issue to public awareness. Not just the kids are suffering, but the parents, as well, because they cannot fulfil their job obligations having to stay home with a sick child. Besides the pneumococcus, there are other resistant bacteria confronting society at large. The tubercle bacillus, which causes tuberculosis, is multidrug resistant and, in some patients, incurable. The gonococcus, the agent of gonorrhoea and a community acquired infection, is now resistant to penicillin, tetracycline, quinolones and some strains show early signs of resistance to cephalosporins. Few if any options remain after the cephalosporins. This is a societal problem. Imagine what's going to happen when we lose our ability to rapidly treat this organism. The staphylococcus can only reliably be treated with vancomycin. To these can be added *Pseudomonas aeruginosa, Acinetobacter* and other bacterial disease agents, all thwarting therapy by resistance. The decade of the 1990s is unique. Resistance is no longer confined to hospital environments, but is now common in community populations worldwide. As important, this crisis is heightened by a lack of new antibiotics developed during the decade.

Approaches to the problem

No novel antibiotic is expected to appear soon, and an increasing number of bacterial infectious agents bear resistance to many if not all antibiotics. We must somehow find a means to reverse the ecological imbalance that has occurred in terms of resistant and susceptible strains. One way is to remove or adjust the selection process so as to allow the susceptible strains to regain their former dominance. As demonstrated above, such reversals are possible and provide the necessary optimism. There still are sufficient susceptible bacteria in our environment which, when given a chance, can return and re-establish the susceptible flora. The crux for reversing and curbing the resistance problem lies in restoring the susceptible microbial flora, whether this is in the intestinal tract, the skin, or elsewhere in the environment. To do this, antibiotic use needs to be more rational. The misconceptions and misunderstandings of antibiotics as miracle drugs without adverse consequences have led to their inappropriate use and prescription. Education of the prescriber and the consumer is critical.

In previous decades the pharmaceutical industry has been able to identify and produce newer and more potent antibacterial agents. However, experience in the present decade indicates that this is no longer true. Discovery has diminished, although encouraging signs are appearing once more (Service 1995). There are now renewed efforts in large pharmaceutical houses and smaller biotechnology companies to discover truly novel drugs. These drugs would be those with no structural relationship to prior antibiotics and thus not intrinsically subject to already existing resistances. This offers one approach towards a solution. Another is to define sufficiently the resistance mechanism and use it to identify novel drugs which can poison or inactivate resistance mechanisms and allow the effective antibiotic to work. This is the basis for the success of the combination of β-lactamase blockers and an effective β-lactam drug, initially introduced as clavulanate and amoxicillin by Beecham Pharmaceuticals. It is this same approach which we are using to restore efficacy to the tetracycline family. Here we are using a semi-synthetic tetracycline to block a drug efflux, allowing a classical tetracycline to enter and stop growth (Nelson et al 1993, 1994).

The control of the antibiotic resistance problem lies in a better understanding of how we use antibiotics. Conditions can be envisioned whereby we encourage the re-emergence of susceptible strains following treatments and the maintenance of the normal susceptible microbial flora between treatments. We need to restore the original microbial balance between susceptible and resistant bacteria — a balance which has been devastatingly altered by the inappropriate and continued application of antibiotics to our environments.

References

Bonten ME, Stobberingh E, Philips J, Houben A 1992 Antibiotic resistance of *Escherichia coli* in fecal samples of two different areas in an industrialized country. Infection 20:258–262

Calva JJ, Sifuentes-Osornis J, Ceron C 1992 Antimicrobial resistance of fecal aerobic gram-negative bacilli in different age groups in a community. Antimicrob Agents Chemother 40:1699–1702

Corpet DE 1988 Antibiotic resistance from food. N Engl J Med 318:1206–1207

DeFlaun MF, Levy SB 1989 Genes and their varied hosts. In: Levy SB, Miller RV (eds) Gene transfer in the environment. McGraw-Hill, New York, p 1–32

Giamarellou H, Antoniadou A 1997 The effect of monitoring of antibiotic use on decreasing antibiotic resistance in the hospital. In: Antibiotic resistance: origins, evolution, selection and spread. Wiley, Chichester (Ciba Found Symp 207) p 76–92

Leistevuo T, Leistevuo J, Osterblad M et al 1996 Antibiotic resistance of fecal aerobic Gram-negative bacilli in different age groups in a community. Antimicrob Agents Chemother 40:1931–1934

Lenski RE 1997 The cost of antibiotic resistance — from the perspective of a bacterium. In: Antibiotic resistance: origins, evolution, selection and spread. Wiley, Chichester (Ciba Found Symp 207) p 131–152

Levy SB 1984 Antibiotic resistant bacteria in food of man and animals. In: Woodbine M (ed) Antimicrobials and agriculture. Butterworths, London, p 525–531

Levy SB 1986 Ecology of antibiotic resistance determinants. In: Levy SB, Novick RP (eds) Antibiotic resistance genes: ecology, transfer and expression. Cold Spring Harbor Press, New York, p 17–29

Levy SB 1992 The antibiotic paradox: how miracle drugs are destroying the miracle. Plenum, New York

Levy SB 1994 Balancing the drug resistance equation. Trends Microb 2:341–342

Levy SB, Fitzgerald GB, Macone AB 1976 Changes in intestinal flora of farm personnel after introduction of tetracycline-supplemented feed on a farm. N Engl J Med 295:583–588

Levy SB, Marshall B, Schluederberg S, Rowse D, Davis J 1988 High frequency of antimicrobial resistance in human fecal flora. Antimicrob Agents Chemother 32:1801–1806

Nelson ML, Park BH, Andrews JS, Georgian VA, Thomas RC, Levy SB 1993 Inhibition of the tetracycline efflux antiport protein by 13-thio-substituted 5-hydroxy-6-deoxy tetracyclines. J Med Chem 36:370–377

Nelson ML, Park BH, Levy SB 1994 Molecular requirements for the inhibition of the tetracyline antiport protein and the effect of potent inhibitors on growth of tetracycline resistant bacteria. J Med Chem 37:1355–1361

O'Brien TF, Stelling JM 1995 WHONET: a program to monitor local and global spread of resistance. APUA Newsletter 13/4:1–6

Roberts MC 1997 Genetic mobility and distribution of tetracycline resistance determinants. In: Antibiotic resistance: origins, evolution, selection and spread. Wiley, Chichester (Ciba Found Symp 207) p 206–222

Service RE 1995 Antibiotics that resist resistance. Science 220:724–727

DISCUSSION

Lenski: The goal of shifting the ecological balance from resistant to susceptible strains of bacteria is clearly an attractive idea. However, how strong is the evidence that when antibiotic usage is relaxed the resistant flora decline? What kinds of rates are we talking about? You gave the example that when you treated yourself with tetracycline it took about three times longer for the resistance to be lost than it did to appear. That struck me as a rather fast rate of disappearance: it suggests there may have been a high cost to resistance for the bacteria.

Bush: In the β-lactamase situation, although ceftazidime resistance can be diminished if you take away the drug, resistance plasmids are maintained in colonizing flora. If the use of ceftazidime is reduced, the number of ceftazidime-resistant isolates will diminish and seem to disappear within a hospital. But it has been demonstrated in Chicago nursing home patients that the plasmids continue to survive in colonizing flora (Wiener et al 1992).

Levy: Thus, although the resistant bacteria are no longer seen as a nosocomial infection, they're still present in the hospital.

Bush: Yes.

Davies: In the tetracycline ingestion experiment, you only analysed tetracycline-resistant organisms of one particular type. You have no idea of the reservoir of tetracycline resistance in the gut flora. Thus it seems to me that the experiment is incomplete and you should do it again using PCR amplification with *tet*-specific primers to find out how long the tetracycline-resistance gene stays around in the gut. I believe that the gene for resistance is going to persist longer than you have shown.

Levy: Tetracycline resistance did not go away. The total tetracycline-resistant *E. coli* flora went back down to what it was before, but it was clearly detectable.

Levin: I once did a similar experiment to that of Stuart, by sampling my own faeces and plating them on antibiotic-free lactose minimal agar and lactose minimal agar containing antibiotics such as streptomycin, ampicillin, kanamycin and tetracycline. In that way it was possible to monitor the frequency of resistant bacteria, even when they were quite rare, in the order of 10^{-5} or less. Before taking tetracycline, the frequency of resistance to the antibiotic was between 10^{-3} and 10^{-2}. One day after I started taking tetracycline, virtually all the bacteria recovered were tetracycline resistant. Moreover, the frequency of resistance to the other antibiotics also increased. Following the termination of treatment, the frequency of resistance to tetracycline and the other antibiotics waned, but continued to oscillate at levels in excess of 10^{-3} for the month or so I sampled for (B. R. Levin, unpublished results).

Levy: There are clearly many other bacteria entering the intestinal flora from the food we eat. Thus there is a lot of mixing with the external flora. A better way to do that experiment would be for me to go on a sterile diet, so I would just be looking at what was happening within my intestinal flora.

Roberts: If you look at the opposite end — the oral cavity — virtually all of us carry tetracycline-resistant α-streptococci, regardless of whether we have had tetracycline or not. Many children who routinely never take tetracycline have tetracycline resistant α-streptococci. One has to go back to the 1960s to find α-streptococci that are susceptible. Many people make the wrong assumption that they are innately resistant, but they have all acquired the *tet* genes. So there are other organisms where you may not get the waxing and waning. We studied bacterial vaginosis in pregnant women, again a group who do not receive tetracycline. Virtually every patient had Tet resistant streptococci and peptostreptococci (Roberts & Hillier 1990). I'm proposing that in streptococci you actually get less fluctuation from susceptible to resistant then you do with *E. coli* in the gut.

Levy: So there's a resident oral flora that persists?

Roberts: Yes. In some of the dental literature, people mistakenly say that the α-streptococci in the oral cavity are intrinsically resistant which is not true; all of them have acquired *tet* genes.

Baquero: That is correct, but the real problem is that it may be too late to react, in the sense that our normal flora is now the normal resistant flora. They have adopted the resistance determinants, perhaps taking advantage of these mechanisms for other functions. One of the key points from your discussion is the concept of a 'resistance gene'. This is a somewhat controversial issue, because many bacteria are normally physiologically insusceptible, or intrinsically resistant. I'm worried by the fate of these intrinsically resistant bacteria in the face of antibiotic pressure. Imagine that we are just looking at potentially pathogenic bacteria: the problem with the multiple antibiotics we are taking to control pathogens is that by their use we are altering our normal bacterial environment. For instance, we are eliminating some of our old lactobacilli and these are replaced by other less 'human adapted' lactobacilli intrinsically resistant to the antibiotics we are using. Perhaps we are changing our normal gut physiology, replacing the bacteria that have been co-selected with us during evolution. Eventually, we are doing something even worse than modifying the pathogenic bacteria — modifying the normal saprophytic bacteria in alliance with human beings through evolution. Who knows what the implications of such changes are for human health?

Summers: Has anybody done any prospective studies on hospital admissions in checking the level of resistance on entry to see what level of resistance indeed does involve subsequent clinical compromise?

Huovinen: We have some results from a study in geriatric units (Leistevuo et al 1996). When someone is treated with an antimicrobial drug, resistant strains will be enriched in this subject and he or she will then excrete these strains to the surroundings.

Levy: You come into hospital with a trace of resistant bacteria. You receive an antibiotic, and resistance frequency rises. Anne Summers is asking: if a patient comes into hospital with 10% resistance, does that level of resistance get them into trouble? I don't know that anyone has done such a prospective study, although many of us have found resistant organisms in the faeces. The frequency probably doesn't matter, because as soon as you start using the antibiotic the numbers rise.

Huovinen: In long-term treatment the patients are colonized in the hospital. We can show that although the level of antimicrobial usage in the ward is very low, patients are still colonized with resistant strains. Antimicrobial treatment is not the only factor.

Cohen: This is a reflection of the underlying problem, which is that we look at only a subset of the microbial flora. Within the greater ecosystem, we're examining just a small part: often just a single pathogen. We often don't know what other species are out there. It is difficult to look at this small microcosm and understand everything that's occurring.

Bush: If we look at the Chicago experience with β-lactamases, the first ceftazidime-resistant β-lactamases appeared in two *Klebsiella* isolates in January 1988. They were not identified again until November 1990 when nursing home patients were then admitted to Chicago hospitals. Resistant *Klebsiella* strains in the hospital were apparently taken back to nursing homes where patients were eventually colonized with *E. coli* with the same plasmids. Species to species transmission was occurring (Wiener et al 1992).

Davies: It's my understanding that we cannot culture all of the organisms in the gastrointestinal tract. The whole point about resistance transfer is that we really don't know where resistance genes are going within the bacterial population. In many cases we don't know what the reservoir is. While we are looking at the bugs that we can grow, we are missing a lot of the microbial ecology of drug resistance.

Noble: It's going to be slightly naïve to look just at one genus, because within a genus you can get quite diverse results. In patients with peritoneal dialysis, the coagulase-negative staphylococci are quite often resistant to three or four antibiotics. In contrast, the coagulase-positive staphylococci are usually sensitive to everything except perhaps penicillin and tetracycline. It may be the case that what is normal on the skin is able to cope with lots of resistant determinants, but what is abnormal on skin can't, unless it's under antibiotic pressure.

Some years ago we showed there are differences between what skin patients have in their nose and what they have on their skin (Noble 1977). What they have on their skin tends to be much more antibiotic resistant even if it's apparently the same strain. There are other factors. For example, many of the penicillinase-producing strains are somewhat more resistant to lipid. We thought this was a rather tidy way of looking at it. It may be that it is actually the skin lipid that is selecting for penicillinase-producing strains, and not the penicillin. We're talking about a resistance determinant as though there's no other DNA on that plasmid or transposon.

Levy: This echoes what Fernando Baquero was saying: can you really call this a 'resistance determinant'? What else might it be doing?

Levin: The basic premise of Stuart Levy's paper is that there is a genetically diverse population containing both bacteria that are resistant and those that are susceptible, and that we should encourage the reservoir of susceptible strains to replace the resistant. On a broader scale, each time antibiotics are used we are increasing the relative frequency of resistance, so that this pristine population you want to replace is going to decline if there is no cost of resistance. Consequently, this reservoir of wonderfully naïve sensitive bacteria would be in a continual state of decline. It seems that already, among the commensal bacteria such as *E. coli*, this sensitive reservoir is already lower than we would like.

Last spring, an undergraduate working in our laboratory, Bassam Tomeh, did a survey of the frequency of resistant bacteria in the faeces of children younger than 30 months in a local day-care centre. He used the lactose minimal-selective plating procedure described above for the egoistic excursion into the comings and goings of my own enteric flora. Bassam's selecting agars contained ampicillin, streptomycin, kanamycin, chloramphenicol and tetracycline. The results, which we are now just analysing, are not optimistic. 15 of the 25 children in the survey were treated with at least one antibiotic during the 3 month sampling period and/or the 3 months before, with one infant being treated with as many as five different drugs during this interval. On average, nearly 50% of the bacteria isolated from these 'treated' infants were resistant to ampicillin, with the entire sample taken from one child being resistant to this antibiotic. Of the total of 13 treated children for whom we had sampled bacteria, resistance to ampicillin was observed in 11. On average, about 25% of the bacteria isolated from the children in this treated subset were resistant to $20 \mu g/ml$ streptomycin. The next most common resistances among the bacteria isolated from the treated children were to kanamycin and tetracycline, about 10% on average. For a few children in the treated sample, the frequency of resistance to these two antibiotics in the bacteria recovered from the faecal samples was substantially higher, as great as 50% and 30%, respectively. Kanamycin and tetracycline resistance, however, was not observed in the flora of the majority of the treated children. On average, the frequency of bacteria resistant to ampicillin and streptomycin in seven untreated children for which we had bacterial samples was no different from that in the treated.

Levy: At the core of the clinician's decision to use antibiotics are sick patients who are not getting better. The attention of the microbiologist is directed to the source of the resistance. Quite clearly some way of combining these aims is needed.

Lerner: We've had an interesting experience in Detroit with MRSA. We are in an unusual situation in that we have a major reservoir of the organisms in the community among intravenous drug users. For over a decade, until recently, the majority of community *Staphylococcus aureus* isolates from intravenous drug-abusing patients as they came into hospital were methicillin-resistant. In the past year or two, the incidence of MRSA in this patient population appears to have declined dramatically, for reasons which are obscure. This decline in resistance is welcome, but we wish we understood it.

Levy: Echoing some of the themes that we've discussed, the change could be the removal of a selective force, or the encouragement of some other organisms which interfere with the resistant organism you have selected.

Baquero: It seems that in several instances where we have a problem with MRSA, things have been getting better, just spontaneously. My impression is that some very clonal bacteria have just got tired of being on top! This may have some genetic background. For instance, one given serotype may be substituted by another in the human population, either because of herd immunity or because the new serotype is resistant to another antibiotic which is also being consumed heavily.

Giamarellou: We have seen the same thing with MRSA: percentage resistance is fluctuating. For instance, after a mean resistance rate of 50% in 1990 the rate went down to 12% in 1992, and then doubled by 1995. I guess that it is resistance in the community that transfers to the hospital, and vice versa. Physicians in the community are concerned about staphylococci and they are aware of the MRSA problem. Therefore they do not use empirically any anti-staphylococcal penicillin in the community for long periods. This fact may explain the fluctuation in MRSA.

Another point that concerns me is that although in Greece people in the community use tons of β-lactams, we have a low rate of *Streptococcus pneumoniae* resistance: only 8% of the intermediate type with a fairly low MIC of 0.25 to 0.5 μg/ml. I cannot explain it.

Witte: Is there real evidence that MRSA has already become part of the colonizing flora in the community? It was my impression that whenever this has been reported there has always been some link back to the hospital. In Germany, the frequency of MRSA doubled from 1990 to 1995. We now have 5% in nosocomial infections. Our community studies have shown that MRSA is still rare among carriers outside hospitals and that we cannot always exclude previous hospital stays.

Roberts: We are currently working with the native population in Alaska, where there is some evidence to suggest that antibiotic resistance has developed *in situ* primarily because they are small communities. For the first 10–12 years there was multidrug resistant *Streptococcus pneumoniae* 6B only in one region of Alaska; now it has been spread all over the state. You will occasionally get another serotype with the same pattern, but this does not seem to spread. There are some factors in the 6B which allow it to be maintained in the community and other factors where it perhaps isn't as good a pathogen, and therefore it may have a little cluster effect but you don't see it maintained for long periods.

Levy: Antibiotics not only select the resistant form of the organism you are trying to treat, but also wreak havoc in the environment. We don't know how large that domino effect is. You cause the resistant organisms to emerge, but they are now in an environment which has also changed. Thus a bacterium that might have been a minor participant in the previous environment, now finds an environment so changed that it can become a major participant.

The antibiotic certainly is a player in the resistance imbalance, but so are the non-target organisms in the environment, many of which we do not know about. We can only look at those things we know. One of the recommendations that I propose should come out of this Symposium is that greater attention should be given to the other organisms being affected by antibiotic use, as well as the factors which cause a change in the levels of resistance which are not linked to antibiotic usage.

References

Leistevuo T, Leistevuo J, Osterblad M et al 1996 Antibiotic resistance of fecal aerobic Gram-negative bacilli in different age groups in a community. Antimicrob Agents Chemother 40:1931–1934

Roberts MC, Hillier SL 1990 Genetic basis of tetracycline resistance in urogenital bacteria. Antimicrob Agents Chemother 36:261–264

Weiner J, Quinn J, Kowalczyk M, Bush K, Rasmussen B, Weinstein RA 1992 Multiple nursing home outbreak of transferable ceftazidime resistant Enterobacteriaceae. 92nd Ann Meet Am Soc Microbiol, New Orleans, LA

Origins, acquisition and dissemination of antibiotic resistance determinants

Julian E. Davies

Department of Microbiology and Immunology, University of British Columbia, 300-6174 University Boulevard, Vancouver, BC, Canada V6T 1Z3

Abstract. Since the introduction of antibiotics in the late 1940s there has been an inexorable propagation of antibiotic resistance genes in bacterial pathogens (and their relatives). This survival phenomenon was first characterized as the appearance of point mutations that altered drug targets, but in the mid-1950s transmissible antibiotic resistance genes were reported in Japan. Since this time both resistance strategies have been used, often in concert. For some types of antibiotic, only resistance by mutation has been identified, for others only resistance by plasmid acquisition. There is conflicting evidence with respect to the presence of antibiotic resistance in bacterial pathogens in the 'pre-antibiotic' era; however, it is likely that the evolution of antibiotic resistance occurred over short periods. Thus, antibiotic resistance genes must be common in the environment, but their derivation remains to be established conclusively. This paper examines the proposals that antibiotic resistance genes originated in the bacterial population, either as *bona fide* resistance genes or genes encoding metabolic functions. In addition, the acquisition of heterologous resistance determinants by different genetic elements, their intergeneric exchange mechanisms, and the possible roles of antibiotics in these processes are discussed. Are there prospects for drug intervention that eliminate or retard these natural evolutionary processes?

1997 Antibiotic resistance: origins, evolution, selection and spread. Wiley, Chichester (Ciba Foundation Symposium 207) p 15–35

The phenomenon of antibiotic resistance presents an unusual aspect of microbial ecology and diversity which has evolved recently, entirely the result of human activity. About 50 years ago, antibiotics were introduced for the treatment of microbial diseases with the expectation that their use would end, once and for all, the threat of infectious diseases. For the microbial population the use of antibiotics created a situation that should have been catastrophic; however, the (then unsuspected) genetic flexibility of bacteria allowed them to survive and even thrive in this hostile environment. What actually happened to the dynamics of the microbial population will never be known, since it is not possible to grow all of the bacterial species and genera that inhabit a given environment; fewer than 1% of microbes are culturable.

In addition, this exciting study in microbial ecology cannot now be conducted, in as much as the earth is very much post-antibiotic.

The proliferation of antibiotic-resistant bacteria under the selective pressures of antibiotic use has led to near-crisis situations in the treatment of infectious diseases. In the case of the enterococci, some hospitals in Europe and North America are plagued with infections that are resistant to all the clinically recommended antibiotics (Moellering 1991, Swartz 1994), there is only one antibiotic available for the treatment of multiply resistant staphylococci in many hospitals worldwide (Green 1994) and antibiotic resistance in pneumococci in the community has increased dramatically (Coffey et al 1995), putting the treatment of infectious diseases back to the pre-antibiotic era. This situation has not developed without warning signals: leading researchers in infectious diseases and microbiology have been emphasizing the potential dangers of resistance since the first use of antibiotics, but the appropriate avoiding action has never been taken. It is now too late. There have been a number of up-to-date reviews on the subject of antibiotic resistance (Trends in Microbiology 1994) and it is not necessary to repeat what has been presented. I propose to focus my comments on several questions concerning the genetic ecology of the development of antibiotic resistance over the last half-century. The analysis must of necessity be retrospective, since there was virtually no attempt to carry out prospective studies at the time when antibiotics were introduced into clinical or agricultural use.

The following points will be discussed in this paper:

(1) What happened to the bacterial population when antibiotics were used, and when and how did resistance develop?
(2) What is the genetic basis of the development of antibiotic resistance?
(3) What are the sources (origins) of antibiotic resistance determinants?
(4) How were heterologous resistance determinants acquired?
(5) In what way(s) was antibiotic resistance disseminated?

The response of the microbial population to the use of antibiotics

The most reliable information on the characteristics of bacteria from the pre-antibiotic era comes from studies of the 'Murray' collection of microbial pathogens that were collected between the years 1914 and 1950. These organisms are completely sensitive to the common antimicrobial agents; even though sulfonamides were introduced into clinical practice in the mid-1930s, the 'Murray' strains do not exhibit resistance to this class of drugs. As was demonstrated by Hughes & Datta (Datta & Hughes 1983, Hughes & Datta 1983), many of the 'Murray' strains carry plasmids and are capable of promoting conjugative transfer. Given that human isolates from the pre-antibiotic era were sensitive to antibiotics, what happened when this bacterial population was exposed to anti-infective agents? Resistance to sulfonamides was first reported in gonococci, pneumococci and streptococci in the early 1940s (Hotchkiss & Evans 1957); although the biochemical nature of the resistance was not characterized at the

TABLE 1   Mutation to antibiotic resistance

Mechanism	Antibiotic
Target alteration	Streptomycin (ribosome)
	Rifampicin (RNA polymerase)
	Fluoroquinolones (DNA gyrase)
	Sulfonamide (DHPS)
	Trimethoprim (DHFR)
Amplification of target enzyme (titration)[a]	Trimethoprim (DHFR)
Amplification of hydrolytic enzyme (inactivation)	Penicillins, cephalosporins (β-lactamases)
Increased efflux ('impermeability')	Fluoroquinolones
Failure to activate pro-drug	Isoniazid (catalase)

[a]Proposed.

time, it was thought most likely to be due to an altered target (the enzyme dihydropteroate synthase) or over-production of the enzyme. Extensive studies by Sköld and co-workers have now given a more complete genetic description of sulfonamide resistance mechanisms (Huovinen et al 1995).

The introduction of streptomycin for the treatment of tuberculosis in 1947 led to the selection of resistant strains due to point mutations in target genes. However, only recently have the mutations been characterized by the use of modern molecular methods (Zhang & Young 1994). The resistant mycobacteria possess streptomycin-resistant ribosomes with altered ribosomal proteins or rRNA (Finken et al 1993). Mutations have also been identified as the cause of resistance to rifampicin (RNA polymerase) (Telenti et al 1993) and macrolides (Meier et al 1994) in mycobacteria and, more recently, to the fluoroquinolone antibiotics (DNA gyrase) in a variety of bacterial pathogens (Ito et al 1994, Guillemin et al 1995). A list of mutationally based resistance phenotypes of clinical significance is shown in Table 1.

More mysterious was the situation that developed in Japan in the mid-1950s during an epidemic of bacillary dysentery (Davies 1995). Multidrug resistance developed rapidly, as has been observed subsequently on the introduction of most 'new' antibiotics (Table 2). On the basis of biochemical mechanism alone, the resistance determinants on R plasmids must have been acquired as intact genes from unidentified sources; there is no possibility that these novel functions could have been derived by mutation within the bacterial host (Table 3). Thus R plasmids, by definition, encode resistance genes acquired from heterologous sources. The biochemical diversity found among the types of resistance mechanisms implies a diversity of origins.

The genetic determinants of antibiotic resistance in bacteria

As has been mentioned above, the first resistant bacterial isolates of clinical significance were the result of mutation. *Mycobacterium tuberculosis* is not known to carry plasmids

TABLE 2   Antibiotic discovery and resistance development

Antibiotic	Discovered	Introduced into clinical use	Resistance identified
Penicillin	1940	1943	1940 (methicillin 1965)
Streptomycin	1944	1947	1947, 1956
Tetracycline	1948	1952	1956
Erythromycin	1952	1955	1956
Vancomycin	1956	1972	1987
Gentamicin	1963	1967	1970

and has no demonstrated gene transfer system. The frequency of mutation to resistance to streptomycin was higher than that found for other bacteria probably because *M. tuberculosis* possesses only one copy of the rRNA gene cluster, making an alteration in a 16S rRNA gene a dominant phenotype. In contrast *Escherichia coli* has seven copies of the rRNA gene cluster and rRNA mutations are recessive, except in rare laboratory-derived instances. In the more clinically frequent situation where the resistant strain carries an R plasmid, the resistance genes are dominant, encoding unique biochemical functions. Mobile structures such as transposons or integrons are often associated with R plasmids and the plasmid may have additional characteristics that favour dissemination, e.g. being itself transposable and often conjugative. The conjugative transposons are most common in bacterial species such as *Bacteroides* (Salyers et al 1995) but have been found in almost all genera.

To summarize, the alternatives for survival presented to the threatened microbial population were either mutation or the inheritance of a novel biochemical function (Table 3). However, the two are not mutually exclusive; mutation leads to 'protein engineering' of an acquired resistance determinant which may expand its substrate range to include semi-synthetic molecules designed to be refractory to the wild-type enzyme; this is nowhere more apparent than in the case of the β-lactamase genes and enzymes (Bush et al 1995). A genetic component responsible for mutational alterations expanding the substrate range of β-lactamases may be the presence of efficient mutator genes in the host and often present on the R plasmid itself. For example, the tester strain used in the 'Ames' test for mutagens, carries a plasmid pKM101 which increases mutation frequencies. The roles of (often) low level changes in antibiotic uptake in the initial development of clinically significant antibiotic resistance have not been well investigated. It is most probable that chromosomal mutations reducing antibiotic uptake through changes in *mar* function (Zhanel et al 1995, Goldman et al 1996) or efflux systems (Lewis 1994, Poole 1994, Takiff et al 1996) were factors in the establishment of an inherited resistance determinant in the host.

TABLE 3 Biochemical mechanisms of antibiotic resistance and their genetic determinants

Mechanism	Examples	Genetic determinants	
		Mutation	Gene acquisition
Reduced permeability	Aminoglycosides	+	+
Pro-drug not activated	Isoniazid	+	
Active efflux	Tetracycline		+
	Fluoroquinolones	+	
Alteration of drug target	Erythromycin		+
	Fluoroquinolones	+	
	Rifampicin	+	
	Tetracycline		+
Inactivation of drug	Aminoglycosides		+
	Chloramphenicol		+
	β-lactams	+	+
'By-pass' inhibited step	Sulfonamides		+
	Trimethoprim		+
Immunity protein	Bleomycin		+
Amplification of target	Trimethoprim	+	
	Sulfonamides	+	
Sequestration of drug	β-lactams	+	+

The sources of inherited resistance determinants

There is now substantial support for the notion that antibiotic resistance determinants were not derived from the current bacterial host of the R plasmid. Perhaps the most compelling evidence for this comes from comparative studies of the genes for β-lactamases and aminoglycoside-modifying enzymes. The two representative phylogenetic trees (Shaw et al 1993, Bush et al 1995) show that, despite similarities within the two protein families, there are considerable sequence differences, and it is not possible to derive a model in which the two classes could have evolved by mutation from common ancestral genes during the past half century. They must have been derived from independent sources, perhaps with the help of natural 'gene shuffling' mechanisms. Resistance genes on R plasmids differ in base composition and codon usage from flanking genes in the host. This is reminiscent of the situation found for genes determining microbial pathogenicity that can be identified as 'islands' of alien nucleic sequence that were inherited as an independent gene cluster from an external source (Blum et al 1994).

TABLE 4   Resistance determinants with biochemical homologues in antibiotic-producing organisms

Antibiotic	Resistance mechanisms
Penicillins	β-lactamases
Cephalosporins	Penicillin-binding proteins
Aminoglycosides	Acetyltransferases
	Phosphotransferases
	Nucleotidyltransferases
Chloramphenicol	Acetyltransferases
Tetracyclines	Efflux system
	Ribosomal protection
Macrolides	Ribosomal RNA methylation
Streptogramins	Esterases
Lincosamines	Phosphotransferases
	Acetyltransferases
Phosphonates	Phosphorylation
	Glutathionylation
Bleomycin	Acetyltransferase
	Immunity protein

Vancomycin resistance in enterococci provides another good example of exogenous inheritance: resistance is determined by a cluster of seven co-regulated genes which are carried on a transposon. The key element is *vanA* which encodes a peptide ligase, leading to the formation of a novel peptidoglycan precursor, UDP-muramyl-tetrapeptide-D-lactate which has low affinity for vancomycin and other glycopeptide antibiotics (Arthur et al 1996, Walsh et al 1996). In wild-type (sensitive) strains, the terminal residue of the precursor is D-alanine, formed by D-ala-D-ala ligase. Phylogenetic comparisons of the known cell wall peptide ligases show that the VanA group falls into a separate and unrelated class, confirming the independent (and unknown) origin of the vancomycin resistance determinants (Evers et al 1996).

Thus one is led to the conclusion that antibiotic-resistance gene clusters of R plasmids were derived from a large and diverse environmental gene pool readily accessible to the microbial population (Levy 1992, Davies 1994). The most obvious source of resistance genes is the organisms that produce antibiotics, since they alone have the mechanistic diversity that is seen in the resistance determinants of clinical isolates of bacteria (Table 4). Confirmation of this comes from the finding that mycobacteria possess tetracycline-resistance determinants identical to those in the tetracycline-producing streptomycete, *Streptomyces rimosus* (Pang et al 1994). None the less, there are gaps in our understanding of the origin of resistance determinants,

TABLE 5   Factors involved in functional inter-microbial gene exchange (acquisition)

In donor	In recipient
Viability	Viability
DNA modification	Competence
Specific functions (*tra, oriT*)	Nucleases
	Restriction/modification
	Integration
	Transcription
	Translation
	Regulation/modulation

e.g. the aminoglycoside nucleotidyltransferases, which have been found only in clinical isolates and have no known relatives. There may be examples of 'housekeeping' functions of resistance genes. Payie et al (1995) have demonstrated that an aminoglycoside acetyltransferase (AAC2'), encoded as a chromosomal gene in *Providencia stuartii*, may play an accessory role in cell wall peptidoglycan formation; other bacterial species are known to possess chromosomal aminoglycoside-resistance genes (Rudant et al 1994). Many bacterial species, including most streptomycetes, contain β-lactamases which are widely distributed in nature, although their 'normal' metabolic function has not been clearly identified. Thus it is clear that antibiotic-resistance determinants could have a number of different genetic sources.

The evolution to functionality of resistance genes in a heterologous host is an important component in the overall development of resistance. Many factors are involved in effective gene exchange between host and recipient (Table 5). Substantial mutational changes are necessary to beget transcription and expression (translational start signals and codon usage, etc.). It is most probable that this tailoring happened in stages as the resistance determinant passed through a cascade of host bacteria. The formation of gene cassettes may have taken place by reverse transcription (Recchia & Hall 1995), a highly mutagenic process that could have contributed to the diversification and adaptation of resistance determinants.

Acquisition

How does a resistance determinant move from the environmental gene pool to a functioning state in a bacterial pathogen? This question seems to have been resolved nicely by the gene cassette/integron model proposed by Hall, Stokes and others (see Hall 1997, this volume). However, in spite of the conceptual simplicity of this process, a number of mechanistic considerations remain to be resolved. For example, how do

TABLE 6   Mechanisms of gene transfer

Mechanism	Transfer
Transformation	DNA/cell
Electroduction	DNA/cell
Ballistics	DNA/cell
Conjugation	Cell/cell
Fusion	Cell/cell
Assimilation	Cell/cell
Liposome-mediated fusion	Micelle/cell
Transduction/transfection	Virus/cell

the gene cassettes form and what is the origin of the integron? To date integrons have been identified only in the *Enterobacteriaceae*, and no similar system of gene acquisition has been identified in other genera. Since there is evidence that at least some R-plasmid-encoded resistance determinants originated in Gram-positive hosts and subsequently transferred to Gram-negative species (Courvalin 1994), the process of gene acquisition in Gram-positive hosts is significant for the evolution of antibiotic resistance.

Dissemination of antibiotic resistance

Two separate aspects of dissemination need to be considered: the passage of resistance genes from the environmental gene pool to clinically relevant hosts, as discussed above, and the horizontal transfer of R plasmids in microbial populations. With respect to the latter, a number of well characterized mechanisms of gene transfer (Table 6) have been identified in the laboratory and it is assumed that these mechanisms operate in nature; however, there may be natural gene exchange systems that are as yet unidentified. In all probability, more than one mechanism is involved in the dissemination of resistance determinants within a bacterial population, since certain species (mycobacteria, for example) appear unable to participate in the processes of gene exchange. In addition to a diversity of plasmid types and antibiotic-resistance mechanisms transferred, R plasmids carry ancillary functions, such as virulence determinants, metal resistance and catabolic genes. These, like antibiotic resistance, may be silent in some hosts and not expressed until transferred to a compatible cytoplasm.

The roles of promiscuous plasmids have been clearly demonstrated in interspecific transfer, and it is generally accepted that broad-host-range transfers played a key role in the dissemination of resistance determinants in the environment (Götz et al 1996). The dissemination of the *tet* genes by conjugative transposons is a prime example (see Roberts 1997, this volume). However, current knowledge of the process of natural

TABLE 7   Evidence for horizontal gene transfer

Direct observation

Use of pure marked isolates in laboratory or nature

    Expression: transcription, translation

    Cryptic: insertion (mutagenic)

Indirect observation

(a) Biochemical

    Identical or similar enzyme activities or properties

    Antibody cross-reaction

(b) Sequence

    Nucleic acid hybridization

    Nucleic acid sequence

    Protein sequence

---

gene transfer (in hospitals or in the intestinal tract) is incomplete. The only component of such events that can be identified is the final product: the R-plasmid-containing strain isolated in the laboratory that is resistant to the antibiotic being employed. The gut and other environments possess diverse collections of bacteria, many of which cannot be cultured in the laboratory. Thus, despite knowledge of gene transfer mechanisms, it is impossible to track the actual pathway of R plasmid dissemination in nature (Table 7). Clearly this is of importance to an understanding of the evolution of resistance genes and R plasmids. Even if it were possible to identify the origin of a specific resistance gene, its migration to its current host involves many gene transfers within a poorly defined microbial population: one organism could mobilize transfer of a plasmid to a different host, the process being mediated by the release of a pheromone produced by yet another microbe! If we are to take laboratory studies of gene transfer at face value, the phylogenetic range of gene exchanges likely includes all living species (Fig. 1) (Amábile-Cuevas & Chicurel 1992). The recent demonstrations of uptake by mammalian cell cultures of DNA of intracellular bacteria are the most extreme examples, raising interesting questions about speciation at the genetic level (Courvalin et al 1995, Sizemore et al 1995).

    The roles of external factors in gene transfers in nature have been little studied; a number of pheromones influencing transfer (and also virulence) have been identified (Salmond et al 1995, Winson et al 1995), and even antibiotics, such as the tetracyclines, actively promote conjugation of resistance elements (Clewell 1993, Stevens et al 1993). The fact that an antibiotic can also promote the transfer of resistance genes (including its own) is a true 'catch-22' situation!

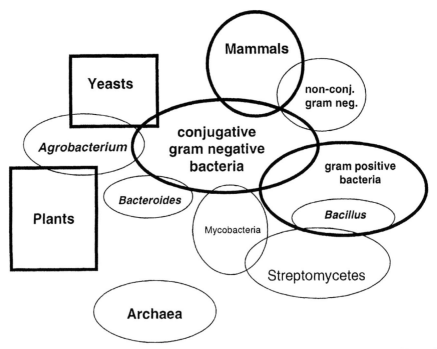

FIG. 1.   The demonstrated range of gene transfer. (Modified from Amábile-Cuevas & Chicurel 1992.)

Conclusion

The problem of antibiotic resistance, its evolution and distribution, is principally one of the genetic ecology of microbial populations. It is evident that there are a large number of contributing factors, some of which are within the power of humankind to control. Whenever an antibiotic is used, bacteria will inevitably develop resistance, either by mutation, gene acquisition, or a combination of the two. It is essential for us to obtain as much information as possible on antibiotic resistance mechanisms and their dissemination and to anticipate the genetic and biochemical forms in which resistance will develop, thereby permitting the design of rational strategies to retard (at least) the inevitable and to prolong the effective lifetime of valuable antimicrobial agents. Our ignorance of many aspects of antibiotic resistance and its development is profound, and until such time as a more substantial knowledge base is generated, medical science can only engage in rearguard actions to defer the spread of resistance.

All this being said, there is one positive aspect of plasmid-determined antibiotic resistance: R plasmids have been the basis of the modern processes of genetic engineering and the biotechnology industry. This may not be a silver lining, but similarly to antibiotic resistance it is a significant feature in the future of humankind.

Acknowledgements

I wish to thank Kevin Chow for making the modifications of the figure and Dorothy Davies for her assiduous efforts in preparation of the manuscript.

References

Amábile-Cuevas CF, Chicurel ME 1992 Bacterial plasmids and gene flux. Cell 70:189–199

Arthur M, Reynolds P, Courvalin P 1996 Glycopeptide resistance in Gram-positive bacteria. Trends Microbiol 4:401–407

Blum G, Ott M, Lischewski A et al 1994 Excision of large DNA regions termed pathogenicity islands from tRNA-specific loci in the chromosome of an *Escherichia coli* wild-type pathogen. Infect Immun 62:606–614

Bush K, Jacoby GA, Medeiros AA 1995 A functional classification scheme for β-lactamases and its correlation with molecular structure. Antimicrob Agents Chemother 39:1211–1233

Clewell DB 1993 Bacterial sex pheromone-induced plasmid transfer. Cell 73:9–12

Coffey TJ, Dowson CG, Daniels M, Spratt BG 1995 Genetics and molecular biology of β-lactam-resistant pneumococci. Microbial Drug Resistance 1:29–34

Courvalin P 1994 Transfer of antibiotic resistance genes between gram-positive and gram-negative bacteria. Antimicrob Agents Chemother 38:1447–1451

Courvalin P, Goussard S, Grillot-Courvalin C 1995 Gene transfer from bacteria to mammalian cells. C R Acad Sci Paris 318:1207–1212

Datta N, Hughes VM 1983 Plasmids of the same Inc groups in Enterobacteria before and after the medical use of antibiotics. Nature 306:616–617

Davies J 1994 Inactivation of antibiotics and the dissemination of resistance genes. Science 264:375–382

Davies J 1995 Vicious circles: looking back on resistance plasmids. Genetics 139:1465–1468

Evers S, Casadewall B, Charles M, Dutka-Malen S, Galimand M, Courvalin P 1996 Evolution of structure and substrate specificity in D-alanine:D-alanine ligases and related enzymes. J Mol Evol 42:706–712

Finken M, Kirschner P, Meier A, Wrede A, Böttger EC 1993 Molecular basis of streptomycin resistance in *Mycobacterium tuberculosis*: alterations of the ribosomal protein S12 gene and point mutations within a functional 16S ribosomal RNA pseudoknot. Mol Microbiol 9:1239–1246

Goldman JD, White DG, Levy SB 1996 Multiple antibiotic resistance (*mar*) locus protects *Escherichia coli* from rapid cell killing by fluoroquinolones. Antimicrob Agents Chemother 40:1266–1269

Götz A, Pukall R, Smit E et al 1996 Detection and characterization of broad-host-range plasmids in environmental bacteria by PCR. Appl Environ Microbiol 62:2621–2628

Green CJ 1994 New antibiotics are needed against *Staphylococci*. Soc Indus Microbiol News 44:231–238

Guillemin I, Cambau E, Jarlier V 1995 Sequences of conserved region in the A subunit of DNA gyrase from nine species of the genus *Mycobacterium*: phylogenetic analysis and implication for intrinsic susceptibility to quinolones. Antimicrob Agents Chemother 39:2145–2149

Hall RM 1997 Mobile gene cassettes and integrons: moving antibiotic resistance genes in Gram-negative bacteria. In: Antibiotic resistance: origins, evolution, selection and spread. Wiley, Chichester (Ciba Found Symp 207) p 192–205

Hotchkiss RD, Evans AH 1957 Genetic and metabolic mechanisms underlying multiple levels of sulphonamide resistance in pneumococci. In: Drug resistance in micro-organisms: mechanisms of development. J & A Churchill, London (Ciba Found Symp 43) p 183–196

Hughes VM, Datta N 1983 Conjugative plasmids in bacteria of the 'pre-antibiotic' era. Nature 302:725–726

Huovinen P, Sundström L, Swedberg G, Sköld O 1995 Trimethoprim and sulfonamide resistance. Antimicrob Agents Chemother 39:279–289

Ito H, Yoshida H, Bogaki-Shonai M, Niga T, Hattori H, Nakamura S 1994 Quinolone resistance mutations in the DNA gyrase *gyrA* and *gyrB* genes of *Staphylococcus aureus*. Antimicrob Agents Chemother 38:2014–2023

Levy SB 1992 Antibiotics, animals, and the resistance gene pool. In: Levy SB The antibiotic paradox: how miracle drugs are destroying the miracle. Plenum, New York, p 137–156

Lewis K 1994 Multidrug resistance pumps in bacteria: variations on a theme. Trends Biochem Sci 19:119–123

Meier A, Kirschner P, Springer B et al 1994 Identification of mutations in 23S rRNA gene of clarithromycin-resistant *Mycobacterium intracellulare*. Antimicrob Agents Chemother 38:381–384

Moellering RC 1991 The enterococcus: a classic example of the impact of antimicrobial resistance on therapeutic options. J Antimicrob Chemother 28:1–12

Pang Y, Brown BA, Steingrube VA, Wallace RJ Jr, Roberts MC 1994 Tetracycline resistance determinants in *Mycobacterium* and *Streptomyces* species. Antimicrob Agents Chemother 38:1408–1412

Payie KG, Rather PN, Clarke AJ 1995 Contribution of gentamicin 2'-N-acetyltransferase to the O-acetylation of peptidoglycan in *Providencia stuartii*. J Bacteriol 177:4303–4310

Poole K 1994 Bacterial multidrug resistance — emphasis on efflux mechanisms and *Pseudomonas aeruginosa*. J Antimicrob Chemother 34:453–456

Recchia GD, Hall RM 1995 Gene cassettes: a new class of mobile element. Microbiology 141:3015–3027

Roberts MC 1997 Genetic mobility and distribution of tetracycline resistance determinants. In: Antibiotic resistance: origins, evolution, selection and spread. Wiley, Chichester (Ciba Found Symp 207) p 206–222

Rudant E, Bourlioux P, Courvalin P, Lambert T 1994 Characterization of the *aac*(6')-Ik gene of *Acinetobacter* sp. 6. FEMS Microbiol Lett 124:49–54

Salmond GPC, Bycroft BW, Stewart GSAB, Williams P 1995 The bacterial 'enigma': cracking the code of cell–cell communication. Mol Microbiol 16:615–624

Salyers AA, Shoemaker NB, Stevens AM, Li L-Y 1995 Conjugative transposons: an unusual and diverse set of integrated gene transfer elements. Microbiol Rev 59:579–590

Shaw KJ, Rather PN, Hare RS, Miller GH 1993 Molecular genetics of aminoglycoside resistance genes and familial relationships of the aminoglycoside-modifying enzymes. Microbiol Rev 57:138–163

Sizemore DR, Branstrom AA, Sadoff JC 1995 Attenuated *Shigella* as a DNA delivery vehicle for DNA-mediated immunization. Science 270:299–302

Stevens AM, Shoemaker NB, Li L-Y, Salyers AA 1993 Tetracycline regulation of genes on *Bacteroides* conjugative transposons. J Bacteriol 175:6134–6141

Swartz MN 1994 Hospital-acquired infections: diseases with increasingly limited therapies. Proc Natl Acad Sci USA 91:2420–2427

Takiff HE, Cimino M, Musso MC et al 1996 Efflux pump of the proton antiporter family confers low-level fluoroquinolone resistance in *Mycobacterium smegmatis*. Proc Natl Acad Sci USA 93:362–366

Telenti A, Imboden P, Marchesi F et al 1993 Detection of rifampicin-resistance mutations in *Mycobacterium tuberculosis*. Lancet 341:647–650

Trends in Microbiology 1994 Special issue: drug resistance. Trends Microbiol 2:341–425

Walsh CT, Fisher SL, Park I-S, Prahalad M, Wu Z 1996 Bacterial resistance to vancomycin: five genes and one missing hydrogen bond tell the story. Curr Biology 3:21–28

Winson MK, Camara M, Latifi A et al 1995 Multiple N-acyl-L-homoserine lactone signal molecules regulate production of virulence determinants and secondary metabolites in *Pseudomonas aeruginosa*. Proc Natl Acad Sci USA 92:9427–9431

Zhanel GG, Karlowsky JA, Saunders MH et al 1995 Development of multiple-antibiotic resistant (Mar) mutants of *Pseudomonas aeruginosa* after serial exposure to fluoroquinolones. Antimicrob Agents Chemother 39:489–495

Zhang Y, Young D 1994 Molecular genetics of drug resistance in *Mycobacterium tuberculosis*. J Antimicrob Chemother 34:313–319

DISCUSSION

Sköld: I would like to comment on trimethoprim resistance mediated by plasmid-borne genes producing drug-resistant dihydrofolate reductases. Almost twenty of these resistance-mediating enzymes have now been observed in bacterial isolates from many parts of the world. When these are arranged together with several other dihydrofolate reductases of both prokaryotic and eukaryotic origin in a phylogenetic tree, five of them are very closely related, but the others are scattered, indicating very different origins.

Davies: Have you any suggestions as to their origin?

Sköld: A likely origin is known for only one resistance determinant, and that is for the *Staphylococcus aureus* resistance enzyme S1, which was shown to be a mutational derivative of the chromosomal *dfr* in *Staphylococcus epidermidis* (Dale et al 1995). Regarding origins, there is also a group of three very closely related enzymes, dfr2a, dfr2b and dfr2c, which are also plasmid-borne. They are completely different and don't fit into the tree at all. These are very inefficient enzymes with high K_ms and monstrously high k_is. The bacteria carrying them are so resistant that they can grow among crystals of trimethoprim in a plate containing a very high concentration of the drug. These enzymes are also different in that they are tetramers of small molecular weight monomers (78 amino acids).

In contrast to the variety of trimethoprim resistance determinants, plasmid-borne sulfonamide resistance by non-drug susceptible dihydropteroate synthase involves only two genes (*sul1* and *sul2*) that are pretty closely related to each other, and are also rather similar to the chromosomal dihydropteroate synthase of *E. coli*. We have looked for others in isolates from all over the world but they are not there, so *sul1* or *sul2* or both account for plasmid-borne sulfonamide resistance in all cases so far studied.

Levy: This is an unusual example of two products in the market dealing with the same pathway, for which resistance to sulfonamide has emerged by only two ways. Nevertheless, sulfonamide resistance is widespread. In contrast, trimethoprim resistance comes in many different packages. What are the origins? We can only deal with what we know, and yet we know that these enzymes don't look like anything we can find elsewhere, but they have got to exist somewhere else — where are they?

Hall: We have been looking at chloramphenicol acetyltransferases (CATs). There are two families of these enzymes that are only related at the superfamily level. One of the CATs is chromosomal in *Agrobacterium* and there's also a closely related open reading frame that's chromosomal in *Pseudomonas* (Bunny et al 1995). We have looked at features such as third codon usage and on this basis it appears that the *Pseudomonas* open reading frame is a *Pseudomonas* gene, but the *Agrobacterium* open reading frame is more likely to have come from *Pseudomonas* (G. D. Recchia & R. M. Hall, unpublished observation). We cloned the *Pseudomonas* open reading frame and found that it confers chloramphenicol resistance but only at a very low level (P. White, W. W. Stokes & R. M. Hall, unpublished observation). The members of this family were probably not originally CATs because they do not acetylate chloramphenicol efficiently, but that doesn't matter in terms of a resistance gene: what matters is whether they can do it well enough to reduce the clinical dose to a level where the bacterium can survive.

Spratt: The timescale of these events is important. It is clear that in many cases the antibiotic resistance genes are homologous to genes in antibiotic-producing microorganisms in the soil. However, they are not *very* similar and I don't think there is any example of a resistance gene found in a pathogen which is virtually identical to a gene found in a producing organism. If these genes moved very recently from soil microorganisms into bacteria they should be virtually identical in nucleotide sequence. This suggests either that antibiotic resistance genes were acquired very recently but we haven't actually found the source yet, or they are much older than that, and they got out of soil microorganisms hundreds of millions of years ago and have been around in other bacteria since then. There are some examples where the latter is true. For example, in all enterobacteria there is a chromosomally encoded β-lactamase and the phylogeny of this gene follows the phylogeny of the enterobacteria (B. G. Spratt, unpublished results). This β-lactamase therefore appears to have been present in the common ancestor of the current enterobacterial species. Why did resistance genes come out of soil microorganisms hundreds of millions of years ago? One thing that strikes me is that if you take an organism such as *E. coli*, it is spending much of its life in the lower intestines of animals, but it is also spending time in sewage and in soil: if we believe the idea that antibiotic genes can protect bacteria from antibiotics produced in the soil, perhaps selection has been occurring for a long time if bacteria are cycling between animals and the soil.

Bush: Certainly, β-lactams are produced by organisms in soil. One of the first bacteria found to produce a monobactam, *Chromobacter violaceum*, also produces a β-lactamase which does not recognize the monobactam as a substrate. Therefore there is some evidence from soil isolates that this is a protection mechanism.

Davies: Surprisingly, many of the resistant organisms have very effective plasmid-borne mutator genes. The plasmids seem to have been constructed with the functions necessary to help in the evolution of a resistance gene, for example to edit for its functional expression in a heterologous host.

Copeland: I remember an article some years ago that talked about the discovery of β-lactamase producers from mummified Egyptian remains about 5000 years old. Did anyone go back and have a look at those and try to match them up with anything around today?

Davies: Not to my knowledge. I believe that antibiotic-producing organisms have been claimed to be present in amber, which makes them old. They would possess antibiotic resistance genes.

Bush: I don't know anyone who has ever seen those mummified isolates but it's a story that keeps being circulated.

Noble: You can push the timescale back if you stop thinking human and think animals, because dermatophytes produce penicillins and fusidanes for example. Hedgehogs almost always have dermatophyte infections and often have penicillin-resistant staphylococci. We have to presume that these resistance genes have been around for millions of years.

Cohen: I think Brian Spratt's hypothesis is fine; the failure previously to recognize resistant strains could simply represent an ascertainment bias. You're not sampling the ecosystems or populations where those organisms exist. Now you change fitness by introducing the antimicrobials into human populations. This will encourage the emergence and recognition of resistant strains in these populations.

Levy: A recurring question seems to be: where are these resistant organisms coming from? They look similar to what we are seeing but they aren't what we are seeing. What are the examples where a resistance determinant from somewhere else has recently moved into some new organism?

Roberts: The oxytetracycline-resistant genes from streptomyces producers have now been found in a number of *Mycobacterium* species causing disease, as well as *Nocardia*. Some of the disease involves the rapid growers which don't necessarily hit immunocompromised patients. In other cases it is related to immunocompromised patient disease which a normal person would not pick up. We found all three of the OTR types: the efflux, the ribosomal protection and the unknown mechanism, in a number of *Mycobacterium* species all of which are tetracycline resistant. We do not see them in those that are susceptible (Pang et al 1994).

Spratt: Do you mean something that is merely homologous or something that is 95% identical?

Roberts: Virtually identical, at very high stringency.

Levy: Another is a tetracycline resistance determinant found in animal species of *Bacteroides* which was found later in human species of *Bacteroides* (Nikolich et al 1994).

Baquero: I would like to comment on Julian's hypothesis concerning the origin of antibiotic resistance in producing organisms. Most bacteria have a vested interest in maintaining the ecology surrounding them. Bacteria producing antibiotics may have an interest in keeping the surrounding stable biological environment in good health. Perhaps they do this by producing resistance genes on plasmids which they then share with their neighbours. Imagine you are parasitizing a leaf and intoxicating it with bleomycin, an antibiotic whose production has been selected for because of its action against foreign, competitive organisms. Why not give the cells you are exploiting a bleomycin resistance mechanism, in order to maintain the ecosystem? Resistance determinants might simply be ecological keys for maintaining a given microcosm.

Davies: Antibiotic activity could just be a serendipitous activity of a number of low molecular weight metabolites produced by bacteria. A number of antibiotics are known to be involved in signalling or quorum sensing.

Summers: Transfer of these resistance genes might take place in 'soil' rather closer to home than outside — i.e. in the intestinal contents. It occurred to me that the organism which is not yet cultivated but which has been identified to cause Whipple's disease is an actinomycete that colonizes the lamina propria of the small bowel.

Levin: As an evolutionary biologist, there is almost no question in my mind that Julian is right that most of the antibiotic resistance genes we are dealing with now, and especially those on plasmids and other accessory elements, were already present long before humans used antibiotics. I also agree that these genes were most likely present in the antibiotic-producing strains of *Streptomyces* and other species. To be sure, there is no way of formally demonstrating that this scenario for the origin of antibiotic resistance is correct. On the other hand, it would be compelling if we could demonstrate that the conditions for evolution of this sort to take place could occur even in trumped-up experiments with contemporary bacteria. The conditions that have to be demonstrated are that (i) as a consequence of their interaction with antibiotic-producing bacteria, selection would favour resistance in otherwise sensitive populations of bacteria, and that (ii) resistance genes can be horizontally transferred from antibiotic-producing microbes to those that are antibiotic-sensitive and then expressed in these strains.

In a recent paper, Pamela Wiener, a postdoc working in my lab, presented evidence that the first of these conditions is met in experimental populations of *Streptomyces griseus* and *Bacillus subtilis* (Wiener 1996). When invading established populations of streptomycin-producing *S. griseus*, streptomycin-resistant *B. subtilis* have a marked advantage over those that are streptomycin sensitive. Her results also demonstrate that streptomycin-producing *S. griseus* have an advantage in protecting established populations from invasion by streptomycin-sensitive *B. subtilis* over non-producing mutants.

Levy: Is your conclusion that this is a clear situation in which the antibiotic production is an event which favours the producer?

Levin: Yes.

Levy: I'm not sure that Julian was actually speaking about that.

Levin: The point that Pam's results address most about Julian's hypothesis is that the conditions for selection of resistance can be met for non-producing bacteria without the use of human antibiotics. I would love to see the other requirement for this hypothesis to be tested: i.e. the horizontal transfer of resistance genes from a producing organism to a sensitive non-producer and the expression of those genes in that sensitive strain.

Lenski: Julian Davies asked about the origins of resistance genes. One of the things that strikes me is that it seems most bacteria can become resistant to antibiotics by mutating the target site, and yet it seems often that the predominant mechanisms of resistance are specific functions that are distinct from simple target alterations, such as detoxication or efflux. Why are these alternative mechanisms of resistance so prevalent? I would put forward the explanation that not only are bacteria selected to become resistant if an antibiotic is part of their environment, but also to do so in a cost-effective way. That is, if there are two different ways of becoming resistant, one of which is to modify the target and the other of which is to pump the antibiotic out of the cell, the bacteria with the cheapest method of resistance will ultimately prevail.

Davies: I may have misled you, because target mutations are not the only type of mutations leading to a resistance phenotype that have been identified. In fact, my guess would be that on exposure to an antibiotic there would be mutation which would affect antibiotic permeability or an efflux system which probably occurs prior to any other mutation leading to antibiotic resistance, in the sense that this gives the organism a chance to survive. Subsequently, other mutational alterations would occur to provide higher levels of resistance. There are many types of mutations which may occur in addition to target mutations that lead to low levels of resistance. Target mutations are not so common in clinical isolates, for example streptomycin resistance in *E. coli*, which occurs at low frequency. They can be isolated with relative ease in the laboratory. Bacterial geneticists thought that mutation to resistance was not going to be a problem in the clinical use of antibiotics because the mutation rate of streptomycin resistance in *E. coli* is 1 in 10^9. As I mentioned, although *M. tuberculosis* is a special case, ciprofloxacin resistance occurs commonly in *Pseudomonas aeruginosa* isolates.

Levy: We are discussing the relative contribution of a target mutation versus an acquired mutation to a resistant phenotype. We often hear that mutations tend to produce organisms that are not very hardy. However, today, many organisms with target gene mutations cause disease. It's the difference between getting a package that's already known to work, versus doing it your own way. In either case you may lose a little bit of competitiveness but survive just enough in a population of a hundred million organisms to sustain a second mutation that improves competitiveness.

Lenski: Part of the equation of selection that we should bear in mind is that there are really two sides to selection: how well a resistance mechanism works when the antibiotic is there, and also how well the bacteria functions in the absence of antibiotic selection. Resistance determinants we see hanging around for a long time will be those that don't cause many harmful side-effects from the standpoint of the bacterium when antibiotic is absent. These side-effects, or the lack thereof, might be just as much a determinant of the long-term success of alternative mechanisms for resistance as their efficacy in avoiding the toxicity of the antibiotic. From the standpoint of the bacterium, it might be a worse compromise to alter a critical target, like a ribosome, than to acquire some discrete new function, such as detoxification.

Davies: But as we said earlier, resistance determinants never go away completely. As far as I am aware, their stability is not related to the biochemical mechanism of resistance.

Cohen: It would be interesting to understand the different frequencies in resistance mechanisms between Gram-positives and Gram-negatives. The organisms are trying to tell us something. Methicillin resistance in methicillin-resistant *S. aureus* (MRSA) is a good example. We have many effective β-lactamases in the same environments as the MRSA, but changes in penicillin binding proteins remain the predominant mechanism of methicillin resistance.

Roberts: Transformation may have some power in that. Many of the penicillin binding protein changes are in organisms that are readily transformable. Most enteric organisms you can transform in the lab, but I don't think it's that easy to transform them naturally.

Levy: What you're saying is what Richard was alluding to: that is, the easiest course of selection may be taken, and that course may be different for Gram-positive versus Gram-negative organisms.

Lerner: Julian mentioned ciprofloxacin, and I wanted to comment on the quinolones. Of course, these didn't exist in nature before their development and introduction into clinical practice, but resistance to them has evolved extremely rapidly. They target a highly conserved 'quinolone resistance determining region' that is homologous in DNA gyrase and topoisomerase IV. A single mutation at a 'hot spot' in either of these targets provides an increment of resistance for survival, and subsequent 'hot spot' mutations produce even greater levels of resistance. It is astonishing how MRSA became resistant to quinolones within months of their introduction into frequent clinical use, so that it is now relatively rare to encounter an MRSA isolate that is susceptible to quinolones. But, despite the frequent association of quinolone resistance to MRSA, the vast majority of methicillin-susceptible *S. aureus* (MSSA) remain susceptible to quinolones, even though it is comparably easy to select for quinolone resistance from both MSSA and MRSA in the lab.

Levy: And yet, as you know, a single mutation in the *gyrA* gene gives only low level resistance: you need additional changes to provide high level resistance. A single mutation in the regulatory *mar* locus also gives you low level resistance. However, that single mutation in *mar* protects the cell from the bactericidal effect of the quinolones (Goldman et al 1996). The mutation creates a large population of bacteria that potentially can mutate to higher level resistance. We do not know whether achieving methicillin resistance protects the cell from other drug-related effects. When you try to select penicillin-resistant *Streptococcus pneumoniae* with penicillin, you cannot achieve very high resistance; but, if you use third generation cephalosporins in selection, you can. The difference is that penicillin is more cidal. This is a key difference among certain antibiotics: those that are lethal and those that leave residual cells. These can further mutate to higher levels of resistance.

Bush: In the case of β-lactams there are interesting things happening that we don't fully understand. In Gram-positives target modification is a predominant resistance mechanism, whereas in Gram-negatives inactivating enzymes and permeability factors seem to be predominant mechanisms.

Huovinen: I would like to raise the question as to whether bacteria can think. For instance, if you look at pneumococcal penicillin resistance produced by mosaic genes, can bacteria assemble different kinds of genes wisely?

Spratt: Rather than building DNA for certain purposes, I think the naturally-transformable pneumococcus is always producing mosaic genes, at a low frequency, by recombinational exchanges with closely-related species. Most of these will be neutral, or deleterious, and will be lost from the population. Occasionally, these interspecies recombinational exchanges result in a phenotype that is strongly selected, as in the case of the mosaic PBP genes that provide increased resistance to penicillin.

Huovinen: To phrase the question slightly differently: can bacteria build DNA for certain purposes?

Hall: It's probably better to turn that round the other way and say, because selective pressure varies or because the environment changes there is an advantage to bacteria in having a certain capacity to modify the arrangement of their genome.

Levy: The machinery for genetic flexibility is there to deal with the changing environment.

Hall: Yes; if the environment is changing, it's advantageous to be able to change.

Davies: It's not the survival of the fittest, it's the survival of what fits.

Summers: I want to make a point about stationary phase variation, which is something even in the classic research organism *E. coli* we're only just beginning to explore. When bugs get out of log phase, where we're so used to studying them, lots of strange things go on that involve genetic rearrangements and perhaps even specific adaptations to immediate environments. That kind of flexibility in any organism provides survivability.

Witte: There is a paper by Bryan Bridges (1996) on adaptative mutations mediated by *mutT*. Under stress the mutational frequency rose by several orders of magnitude.

Levy: Even without known mutator genes, bacteria in stationary phase show different mutation rates and kinds of mutations from those in logarithmic phase. The mutation rates of bacteria in stationary phase could be enormously higher.

Threlfall: I do not think that we have fully taken into account the actual spread of the organism itself. In Gram-negative pathogens such as *Salmonella*, we see a strain becoming resistant and then spreading. The acquisition of resistance itself may be just one small event in that, but it is the dissemination of the strain which is quite critical. In Britain we are currently experiencing an epidemic of multiresistant *Salmonella typhimurium*. This is being caused by the spread of a small number of closely related strains in food animals, particularly bovines but also in poultry, pigs and sheep. However, it is important to emphasize that it is fundamentally one strain that is spreading.

In addition, we are now seeing the chromosomal integration of resistance in a significant proportion of multiresistant *S. typhimurium*. The same is also true for *Shigella dysenteriae* type 1 in developing countries, where in many instances multiresistance in this organism is chromosomal.

Levy: Were these genes previously carried on plasmids that have become chromosomally located?

Davies: They are insertions.

Skurray: As I shall describe in my paper (Skurray & Firth 1997, this volume), there are specific examples in multiresistant strains of *Staphylococcus aureus* where entire plasmids have integrated into the chromosome to give chromosomal tetracycline or aminoglycoside resistance. Consequently, the chromosome of *S. aureus* is now developing as a major contributor to multiresistance in these strains. As such this provides a very stable source of resistance genes.

Levy: We are seeing changes which we can actually pinpoint to the antibiotic era. Marilyn Roberts has detected tetracycline resistance genes in *Mycobacterium* where they were never detected before (Roberts 1997, this volume). We see whole plasmids integrating into chromosomes. It seems there are certain events which we can document now. In some instances we can say that this event has occurred within the period of widespread antibiotic use.

Hall: The multidrug resistant strains and the resistance transfer factors (plasmids), such as NR1 (also known as R100) that they carry emerged in a very short time after the introduction of antibiotics. NR1 has four antibiotic resistance genes and a mercury resistance determinant on it, and it seems rather unlikely that each of those genes would evolve and then get themselves set up to be mobile all in less than 10 years. My view of what happened is that the genes and plasmids were already out there and they got into the clinical situation by chance and selection. One actually sees the same configuration of genes subsequently turning up all round the world. So, we could argue that they were the first through the eye of the needle and had the chance to grow to such a large population within the clinical environment, that a second comer would have to be pretty competitive to ever overtake them. Consequently, they became dominant not because they were the best genes but because they got the front running. You could argue the same for TEM, that it is the dominant β-lactamase in Gram-negatives, not necessarily because it's the best β-lactamase but because it was the first that got into the new niche. There are many other β-lactamase resistance genes but TEM continues to dominate.

Lerner: The report in 1983 of a β-lactamase encoded by a transferable plasmid in enterococci seemed to portend even greater resistance to ampicillin in these organisms, as the β-lactamase would be selected and disseminated with the plasmid (Murray & Mederski-Samoroj 1983). For reasons that remain obscure, the prevalence of β-lactamase in enterococci has remained minimal. Why hasn't it spread?

Levy: The presence of the β-lactamase in *Enterococcus* is of interest not only because it hasn't increased noticeably, but also because of its origin, i.e. the staphylococcus. One could question why it took so long for the enterococcus to pick up the staphylococcal β-lactamase which has been recognized for decades. In fact, it does not seem to work very well in the enterococcus: the enzyme is bound to the membrane and is not excreted. A better construct of the gene has not appeared — perhaps selection is not adequate.

References

Bridges B 1996 Elevated mutation rate in mutT bacteria during starvation: evidence for DNA turnover. J Bacteriol 178:2709–2711

Bunny KL, Hall RM, Stokes HW 1995 New mobile gene cassettes containing an aminoglycoside resistance gene, *aaca7*, and a chloramphenicol resistance gene, *catb3*, in an integron in pbwh301. Antimicrob Agents Chemother 39:686–693

Dale GE, Broger C, Hartman PG et al 1995 Characterization of the gene for the chromosomal dihydrofolate reductase (DHFR) of *Staphylococcus epidermidis* ATCC 14990: the origin of the trimethoprim-resistant S1 DHFR from *Staphylococcus aureus*? J Bacteriol 177:2965–2970

Goldman JD, White DG, Levy SB 1996 The multiple antibiotic resistance (*mar*) locus protects *Escherichia coli* from rapid cell killing by fluoroquinolones. Antimicrob Agents Chemother 40:1266–1269

Murray BE, Mederski-Samoroj B 1983 Transferable β-lactamase. A new mechansism for *in vitro* penicillin resistance in *Streptococcus faecalis*. J Clin Invest 72:1168–1171

Nikolich MP, Hong G, Shoemaker NB, Salyers AA 1994 Evidence for natural horizontal transfer of *tetQ* between bacteria that normally colonize humans and bacteria that normally colonize livestock. Appl Env Microbiol 60:3255–3260

Pang Y, Brown BA, Steingrube VA, Wallace RJ Jr, Roberts MC 1994 Tetracycline resistance determinants in *Mycobacterium* and *Streptomyces* species. Antimicrob Agents Chemother 38:1408–1412

Roberts MC 1997 Genetic mobility and distribution of tetracycline resistance determinants. In: Antibiotic resistance: origins, evolution, selection and spread. Wiley, Chichester (Ciba Found Symp 207) p 206–222

Skurray RA, Firth N 1997 Molecular evolution of multiply-antibiotic-resistant staphylococci. In: Antibiotic resistance: origins, evolution, selection and spread. Wiley, Chichester (Ciba Found Symp 207) p 167–191

Wiener P 1996 Experimental studies on the ecological role of antibiotic production in bacteria. Evol Ecol 10:405–421

The relationship between erythromycin consumption and resistance in Finland

Pentti Huovinen, Helena Seppälä, Janne Kataja, Timo Klaukka and the Finnish Study Group for Antimicrobial Resistance

Antimicrobial Research Laboratory, National Public Health Institute, PO Box 57, SF-20521 Turku, and Social Insurance Institution, Helsinki, Finland

Abstract. Because the discovery of new antimicrobial agents cannot be expected in the near future, we will have to manage with the antimicrobials currently available at least for the next decade or two. Therefore, attempts to prevent development of antimicrobial resistance are of major importance. The relationship of local antimicrobial consumption and antimicrobial resistance has been shown in many hospital studies but not in the community, even though this is where most antibiotics are used. At the beginning of 1990s, erythromycin resistance in group A streptococci increased rapidly in Finland. The geographical variations found led to a nationwide study of the possible relation between local erythromycin consumption and variations in erythromycin resistance in the community. Erythromycin resistance was found to be significantly ($P = 0.006$) linked to local consumption of erythromycin. In further experiments, we found that a new erythromycin resistance phenotype belonging to the T4 serotype was spread over the whole country; 83% of the erythromycin-resistant isolates were of this new phenotype in 1994. In 1991, recommendations were given to reduce use of erythromycin in Finland. Following these recommendations, macrolide consumption decreased by 40% from 1991–1994. Studies are now in progress to evaluate the effect of this reduction on erythromycin resistance of group A streptococci.

1997 Antibiotic resistance: origins, evolution, selection and spread. Wiley, Chichester (Ciba Foundation Symposium 207) p 36–46

There are three principal ways to resist infectious diseases. Two of those are preventive: hygienic measures and vaccinations. In the community it is difficult, if not impossible, to implement strict hygienic measures effectively. Although vaccinations have changed enormously the spectrum of infectious diseases, effective vaccines against many major bacterial pathogens have not yet been developed.

The third way, antimicrobial therapy, is used for the treatment of existing infections, or prophylactically. Antimicrobials are generally safe to use and easy to administer — in effect, a potentially fatal disease can be treated with a few pills. It has been said that antimicrobial agents are too good to be true. They are real miracle drugs (Levy 1992).

36

Antimicrobials have now been in use for more than 60 years. During this period a tremendous selection pressure has been exerted on human bacterial pathogens. If we look the history of antimicrobial agents, development of bacterial resistance against antimicrobial agents has been an expected but rather unpredictable phenomenon.

Today, the worldwide increase of antimicrobial resistance poses a serious clinical problem (Neu 1992). Because the discovery of new, problem-solving antimicrobial agents cannot be expected within the next 10–20 years, we will have to manage with the antimicrobials currently available. Consequently, attempts to prevent development of antimicrobial resistance are of major importance.

The relationship between antimicrobial consumption and antimicrobial resistance has been shown in many hospital studies, but not convincingly in the community, even though this is where the majority of antibiotics are prescribed. For example, in Finland 88% of antimicrobial treatment is administered to outpatients.

Group A streptococcus (*Streptococcus pyogenes*) shows a prevailing high pathogenicity. During the last decade a resurgence of severe forms of disease caused by this pathogen has taken place in different parts of the world. Fortunately, group A streptococci worldwide are still susceptible to penicillin, which has remained the drug of choice. In Finland, however, a worrying increase in resistance to erythromycin, which is widely used to treat penicillin-allergic patients, was noted in the late 1980s/early 1990s. The frequency of erythromycin resistance among isolates of group A streptococci from pharyngeal and pus samples increased from approximately 5% in 1988–1989 to 13% in 1990. Among isolates from blood cultures the resistance rate increased from 4% in 1988 to 24% in 1990 (Seppälä et al 1992). In the preceding few years, consumption of erythromycin in Finland had nearly tripled.

After the nationwide increase of erythromycin resistance in group A streptococci was first noted, it was thought that the only way to control this clinically important resistance problem was to restrict the use of erythromycin and, due to cross-resistance, also other, newer macrolides (Seppälä et al 1992). Therefore, national recommendations were given to reduce the use of these agents in the treatment of outpatients (Huovinen & Klaukka 1991, Huovinen 1992).

In addition to the recommendations to reduce use of macrolides, we started a nationwide study with three branches:

(1) The geographical variations of the erythromycin resistance found led to a nationwide study of the possible relation between local erythromycin consumption and erythromycin resistance in the community.
(2) A nationwide study was conducted to follow the effect of the selected antimicrobial policy in the pattern of erythromycin resistance.
(3) We also began to study clonal variations of group A streptococci collected from different parts of the country to reveal the possible spread of a single clone of *Streptococcus pyogenes* in Finland.

Methods

Macrolide consumption

Macrolide consumption figures are obtained from the Finnish Statistics on Medicines, published by the Social Insurance Institution and the National Agency for Medicines. Data are available annually and are presented in terms of defined daily doses (DDD)/ 1000 inhabitants per day. For special purposes it is possible to get permission to obtain precise local consumption figures.

Bacterial susceptibility testing

Reliable susceptibility testing is a cornerstone of this type of study. We have tried to minimize possible errors in erythromycin susceptibility testing of group A streptococci (Nissinen et al 1995). For group A streptococci this task is rather easy because of the clear difference in minimum inhibitory concentration (MIC) distribution between the resistant and susceptible isolates.

The second task is to collect bacterial strains from the area studied. For this purpose we have built the FiRe network, the Finnish Study Group for Antimicrobial Resistance. A total of 25 major clinical microbiological laboratories from each part of the country have participated.

Typing of group A streptococci

There are currently three different phenotypes of erythromycin-resistant group A streptococci. These macrolide–lincosamine–streptogramin resistance (MLS resistance) phenotypes can be identified by different behaviour in the induction test, where erythromycin and clindamycin discs are placed close to each other. In inducible-type MLS resistance, clindamycin resistance is induced by erythromycin and is seen as a flattened zone of inhibition around the clindamycin disc. Another earlier known type of resistance is constitutive-type resistance, where isolates are resistant to both erythromycin and clindamycin. Among Finnish erythromycin-resistant group A streptococci a third type, so-called 'novel-type' erythromycin resistance, has also been found; these strains are resistant to erythromycin but susceptible to clindamycin and do not show any induction of clindamycin resistance (Seppälä et al 1993).

Typing of group A streptococci is classically based on serotyping. In addition, we have introduced a restriction endonuclease assay (REA) and random amplified polymorphic DNA analysis (RAPD) in our laboratory (Seppälä et al 1994a,b).

Results and discussion

Relationship between local consumption of erythromycin and erythromycin resistance

In 1992, we studied more than 10 000 group A streptococcal isolates from 206 health authority areas in Finland (Seppälä et al 1995). This definitive analysis, comprising 92%

of all health authority areas in the country, further confirmed that in a given area, use of erythromycin had affected significantly the level of erythromycin resistance in group A streptococci. Logistic regression analysis showed that in 1991 the proportion of these outpatient isolates resistant to erythromycin increased significantly ($P = 0.006$) with increasing local erythromycin consumption. Interestingly, resistant throat isolates occurred most often among children younger than 5 years. In this age group the use of erythromycin was highest.

There are several factors that influence antimicrobial resistance of bacteria in the community. Antimicrobial consumption is perhaps only one selective force. Characteristics of the microorganism and the presence of human and possibly other reservoirs of resistance organisms or resistance genes certainly also have an impact. In addition, transport networks and social factors (day care centres, schools, etc.) that promote transfer of microbes between humans are difficult to standardize.

Our discovery of the relationship between erythromycin resistance and erythromycin consumption was somewhat fortuitous: perhaps the only period in which association between antimicrobial consumption and resistance can be detected is when resistant pathogens are rapidly increasing in the community but have not yet emerged in all parts of the country. If resistance levels are already high, this association is more difficult to study properly.

Decrease of erythromycin consumption

The attempt to reduce erythromycin use in 1991–92 was based on three different measures. First, several months before publishing the recommendations to reduce erythromycin use we informed major erythromycin-marketing pharmaceutical companies in Finland. In early autumn 1991, the marketing strategies for the next year were in a planning phase and we wanted the pharmaceutical industry to be aware of the situation.

Second, we published an editorial in the *Finnish Medical Journal* in the beginning of December 1991 (Huovinen & Klaukka 1991). The aim of this article was to encourage reduced use of erythromycin wherever and whenever possible. This message was boosted with a press release when our original article in the *New England Journal of Medicine* was published in January 1992 (Seppälä et al 1992).

Third, a few months later an article was published in the *Finnish Medical Journal* concerning indications of erythromycin use (Huovinen 1992).

These measures were very well received. Concerning the drug marketing, the pharmaceutical industry pointed out the same facts as mentioned in our publications. Following the recommendations, macrolide consumption in Finland decreased by 40% between 1991 and 1994 (Table 1). This was replaced by an increase in the use of doxycycline and first and second generation cephalosporins — the total consumption of antimicrobial agents did not change.

In 1995, however, consumption of macrolides was increasing again (in 1994–95 from 1.38 to 1.88 DDD/1000 inhabitants per day) due to more effective marketing of

TABLE 1   Macrolide consumption in Finland 1990–95

Year	Macrolide consumption[a]	Percentage change compared with previous year
1990	2.56	—
1991	2.56	±0%
1992	1.48	−42%
1993	1.56	+10%
1994	1.38	−11%
1995	1.88	+36%

[a]Defined daily dose/1000 inhabitants per day.

newer macrolides. This has happened even though our recent recommendations for antimicrobial use in outpatients do not favour the use of macrolides as a first-line drug in respiratory tract infections other than pneumonia (Huovinen & Vaara 1995).

Studies are now in progress to evaluate the effect of the reduction of macrolide usage on erythromycin resistance of group A streptococci during the period 1992–95.

Typing of the erythromycin-resistant group A streptococci

Our first studies found no predominance of certain serotypes among erythromycin-resistant group A streptococci (Seppälä et al 1992). Later we found that a new, non-inducible phenotype of erythromycin resistance was widespread (Seppälä et al 1993). These isolates were resistant to erythromycin but susceptible to clindamycin (clindamycin resistance could not be induced) and accounted for 38% of the resistant isolates. This finding lead us to study further possible clonality of erythromycin-resistant group A streptococci.

In 1994 we studied 695 erythromycin-resistant group A streptococci; of these, 83% were of the new phenotype. Closer analysis showed that 91% of the isolates that belonged to the new phenotype were of the T4 serotype. In addition, 75% of the isolates of the classical inducible type of resistance belonged to the T28 serotype. RAPD and REA studies showed that the majority of the resistant T4 serotype isolates were highly homologous. It is possible that at least part of the increase of erythromycin resistance in Finland is due to just a few clones of group A streptococcus. Further analysis is in progress.

In conclusion, we now are living in a very interesting phase in Finland. We have shown that the occurrence of erythromycin-resistant group A streptococci is linked to increased local use of erythromycin. Second, this phenomenon is at least in part due to the spread of one single clone of erythromycin-resistant group A streptococcus. Third, the decrease of erythromycin and macrolide consumption will serve as a unique opportunity for us to study the effect of planned antibiotic policy on resistance levels of a pathogenic bacterium.

Acknowledgement

This study was supported by the Sigrid Juselius Foundation.

References

Huovinen P 1992 Milloin erytromysiiniä ja mitä sen sijaan? (Engl transl: When to use erythromycin and how to replace it?) Suom Lääkäril 47:13

Huovinen P, Klaukka T 1991 Erytromysiinin käyttöä vähennettävä. (Engl transl: Use of erythromycin had to be reduced.) Suom Lääkäril 46:32–41

Huovinen P, Vaara M 1995 Avohoidon mikrobilääkkeet. (Engl transl: Use of antimicrobial drugs in the community.) National Agency for Medicines and KELA, Forssa

Levy SB 1992 The antibiotic paradox: how miracle drugs are destroying the miracle. Plenum, New York

Neu HC 1992 The crisis of antibiotic resistance. Science 257:1064–1073

Nissinen A, Seppälä H, Huovinen P, Finnish Study Group for Antimicrobial Resistance (FiRe) 1995 Detecting erythromycin resistance in *Streptococcus pyogenes*: reliability of the disk diffusion method and the breakpoint susceptibility testing method. Scand J Infect Dis 27:52–56

Seppälä H, Nissinen A, Järvinen H et al 1992 Resistance to erythromycin in group A streptococci. N Engl J Med 326:292–297

Seppälä H, Nissinen A, Yu Q, Huovinen P 1993 Three different phenotypes of erythromycin-resistant *Streptococcus pyogenes*. J Antimicrob Chemother 32:885–891

Seppälä H, He Q, Österblad M, Huovinen P 1994a Typing of group A streptococci by random amplified polymorphic DNA analysis. J Clin Microbiol 32:1945–1948

Seppälä H, Vuopio-Varkila J, Österblad M et al 1994b Evaluation of methods for epidemiologic typing of group A streptococci. J Infect Dis 169:519–525

Seppälä H, Klaukka T, Lehtonen R, Nenonen E, Finnish Study Group for Antimicrobial Resistance (FiRe), Huovinen P 1995 Outpatient erythromycin use: link to increased erythromycin resistance in group A streptococci. Clin Infect Dis 21:1378–1385

DISCUSSION

Witte: How frequent is serotype T28 among *Streptococcus pyogenes* in general? Also, have you confirmed your assumption of the clonal spread of a particular strain by molecular typing?

Huovinen: We haven't published those results yet. Among erythromycin-susceptible throat isolates, about 30% are of the T28 serotype, but only 16% are of the T4 serotype.

Lerner: Although in the USA we don't have an organized healthcare system as you do in Scandinavia, we try to encourage appropriate use of antibiotics by continuing education of physicians and education of patients via the media. After a recent talk to a state convention of family physicians I was especially pleased when several of the physicians told me that when their patients come to see them now they often refuse antibiotics because they have heard on television about the resistance problem. Consequently, I think we are getting the message through and people are often more receptive than we give them credit for. I've given talks to physicians for many years regarding the two-edged sword of antibiotics, and it's only recently that they have begun to be interested. I think the advent of penicillin resistance in *Streptococcus pneumoniae* is largely responsible for this. Although we have been talking for years about the horrendous multiresistant Gram-negatives we have in the hospital, the concern of physicians about the *S. pneumoniae* problem has really brought home to them the message of resistance.

Bennish: However, increased awareness on the part of physicians can be a mixed blessing because the publicity about resistance has in part made physicians think they have to go the next level up. The situation in the USA may be different from that of Scandinavia where there's this great social cohesiveness: paediatricians in the USA may think lawyers first and community interest second.

Giamarellou: What did you replace erythromycin with? Did you use penicillin or did you educate the people that their diseases were probably viral? Is clarithromycin prescribed in Finland? At least in Greece, this has almost replaced erythromycin.

Huovinen: Clarithromycin has very low sales figures in Finland. Azithromycin and roxithromycin are the predominant macrolides at the moment. I would stress that our instructions are not orders, rather recommendations. The physician has the final decision in every case. For treatment of tonsillitis, our recommendations are that microbial diagnosis is carried out, and penicillin is the drug of choice. 80% of cases are treated with penicillin. The second choice is one of the first generation cephalosporins. According to the results of the susceptibility test, it is permissible to use macrolides if they are needed or if the local erythromycin resistance rate is low.

Giamarellou: How often do you administer oral Pen V?

Huovinen: The recommendation is 1–1.5 million units twice or 1 million units three times a day.

Sköld: How large a fraction of the total macrolide consumption was given on the specific diagnosis of *Streptococcus pyogenes* infection?

Huovinen: We don't have indication-based studies from before 1995, but I assume it was 20–30%.

Levy: You mentioned that mycoplasma was the target organism.

Huovinen: Yes, mycoplasma was a reason for using macrolides, but people thought that every disease was caused by mycoplasma and that was given as a justification for using macrolides.

Sköld: There might be an over prescription of macrolides by doctors because of the fear of hypersensitivity of patients to penicillin, the risk of which may well be exaggerated.

Huovinen: That's true. 10% of Finnish people say that they are hypersensitive to penicillin, but the real figures are lower — about 1–2% or even less.

Lipsitch: What has happened with resistance to the antibiotics you substituted for erythromycin?

Huovinen: In these indications the most commonly used drugs are penicillin and the first generation cephalosporins. We haven't found any changes in resistance for these.

Levy: Do you have any tetracycline-resistant *S. pyogenes*?

Huovinen: Yes, but not many.

Roberts: We've had a few out of Harborview Hospital, the county facility in Seattle, and most of the time they are resistant to both tetracycline and erythromycin. The resistance genes are moveable, on conjugative elements.

Huovinen: Remember that tetracycline was used in other indications apart from tonsillitis.

Levy: *S. pyogenes* has always represented a beacon of susceptibility and now we see strains resistant to macrolides and tetracycline. Clearly, with time, even these have succumbed.

Copeland: The linkage between antibiotic usage and decreased susceptibility is interesting, particularly with regard to macrolides.

Until 1993 macrolide usage in the USA was fairly static at around 300 metric tonnes of pure active per annum. Following the introduction of 'newer' macrolides, the consumption had increased by a third by 1995. This level of growth was the largest of any antibiotic class. Against this background will the susceptibility of respiratory tract pathogens change?

Huovinen: There are areas where macrolides are very heavily used with little development of resistance. However, once the resistance genes arise among bacterial pathogens, rapid development of resistance is likely to be seen.

Levy: You define your usage on the basis of the individual. However, these individuals could be crowded into some of the cities and rather dispersed in other areas. Have you looked at the density of antibiotic use on a person per space basis, to see how proximal individuals are to each other in terms of looking at the correlation between antibiotic use and resistance?

Huovinen: We tried to take this into account, but we couldn't find any effective statistical method to examine it with.

Davies: To what extent are macrolides used for agricultural purposes in Finland?

Huovinen: Almost none.

Davies: You don't use tylosin, or anything like that?

Huovinen: Tylosin is used, if you consider that to be a macrolide.

Davies: Tylosin is a macrolide and bacteria resistant to tylosin will also be resistant to other macrolides.

Huovinen: Remember that group A streptococcus is more commonly a human pathogen.

Levy: It is easier to show a relationship between animal use of antibiotics and human health problems if the pathogen is shared. It is also true that antibiotics are being given to large populations of animals where people are also present. So you have no idea what influence the antibiotic has on bacteria associated with people even if the organism *per se* is not shared by both groups. It is the antibiotic which is selective.

Baquero: As far as animals are concerned, the only risk I remember is from cats, which are frequently carriers of *S. pyogenes.* I don't know whether cats are usually treated with tylosin, other macrolides or streptogramins.

Summers: With this regimen you appear to have decreased erythromycin resistance by a factor of two. What effect have you seen on treatment failures?

Huovinen: We haven't measured treatment failures after we instituted these recommendations to reduce macrolide use. The resistant strains were causing treatment failures pre-1992. Today, it is difficult to study this because macrolides are no longer used in infections caused by group A streptococci.

Summers: But you are still using erythromycin on 40% of your people.

Huovinen: Yes, but in other indications — not in tonsillitis or skin infections. In 1995, macrolides were used at the rate of 1.8 defined daily doses/1000 inhabitants per day.

Baquero: You have a double selection, with some strains having the 23 S rRNA methylase-mediated resistance (high level resistance to macrolides) and then the new mechanism of efflux, functionally — but not genetically — resembling MsrA from *Staphylococcus* (low-level resistance).

Huovinen: PCR with primers for known erythromycin resistant genes has been unsuccessful in isolates with the new resistance phenotype.

Baquero: We have exactly the same type of phenotype in viridans streptococci. Have you looked at viridans streptococci as a reservoir of this type of gene? This might help to explain how the dissemination has been taking place. On the other hand, in order to ascertain the value of your antibiotic policy, have you considered looking at a control country? If you were to cross the border to Russia, you could look at pharyngeal colonization there, where they haven't taken any measures to decrease erythromycin resistance.

Huovinen: We have been involved with the Russian resistance problems quite a bit, and I suspect they are not eager to study group A streptococci when multiresistant TB and diptheria are their biggest problems.

Witte: I remember that at the end of the 1970s in the St Petersburg area, macrolide-resistant *S. pyogenes* isolates had already been found and were characterized by Dr Totoljan. At the same time we hadn't seen this in other Eastern European countries.

Huovinen: Erythromycin resistance was a relatively rare phenomenon among group A streptococci before 1988. The resistance levels were about 1–2%.

Levy: Does anyone have figures for other countries?

Giamarellou: We don't have a problem in Greece.

Baquero: We have a problem in Spain, particularly in the north. In Basque country, resistance levels are about 15%.

Huovinen: In Italy resistance levels have been as high as 30–35% and in Sweden about 5%, depending on the areas studied.

Levy: A unique advantage in Finland is that the population is fairly homogeneous, and the different areas are rather distinct with very different frequencies not only of use but also of resistance. When you showed the reduction in resistance you combined the data from all areas. Was there a more rapid change in areas that were less densely populated?

Huovinen: No. In the southern part of Finland it's coming down, but in Lapland levels are peaking. The resistance percentage at the moment is much higher in Lapland.

Levin: We have developed a model to examine the relationship between the incidence of treatment and the frequency of resistance (Levin et al 1997). In this model there is an array of hosts who are treated with an antibiotic T times per year. We assume that once treated, the frequency of resistant bacteria in the hosts ascends to unity. In untreated hosts, following the termination of treatment the frequency of resistant bacteria declines at a rate proportional to a selection coefficient, s $(0 < s < 1)$. Hosts shed their bacteria into the common environment and receive bacteria from that common environment at rates f and g, respectively. At equilibrium, the frequency of resistance depends critically on the intensity of selection against the resistant type, s, and the incidence of treatment. For example, with $f = 0.05$, $g = 0.005$ and treatment once a year, for $s = 0.01$ and $s = 0.04$, the equilibrium frequencies of resistance predicted by our simulations are approximately 0.54 and 0.20, respectively. If we reduce the incidence of treatment to once every second year, the corresponding equilibrium frequencies are 0.30 and 0.10. A selection coefficient of $s = 0.01$ is in essence only a 1% lower growth rate for the resistant bacteria relative to the sensitive ones.

Lenski: Bruce Levin's model is simple and elegant. However, the assumption that the frequency of resistant bacteria in a treated host goes to one makes sense only if one considers a commensal population. In the case of a pathogen, it seems to me that there should be another outcome: successful treatment that eliminates the population without the appearance of resistance. If that were true in, say, 90% of the cases, then it would knock the overall equilibrium frequency of resistant bacteria in the population down by an order of magnitude.

Levin: You are quite right, Richard: this model is intended mainly for commensal bacteria that are picked up from a common pool, rather than directly transmitted from symptomatic hosts bearing those bacteria as in the case of tuberculosis. Rustom Antia has developed an epidemiological compartment-like model for the latter situation. The results obtained with that model are very different from those from our model of commensal bacteria. There, you have a threshold treatment level beyond which the infected host population is dominated by hosts bearing the resistant bacteria, and below which the resistance is rare.

Huovinen: I will explain how we intend to proceed. There are about 3.3 million antimicrobial treatments annually in Finland for a population of about 5 million. About 2.5 million of these courses are actually supported by the state insurance company, so all these individual case data are on computer. In the FiRe network we can collect individual data on different bacteria, because we have hundreds of thousands of susceptibility tests in Finland annually. We could combine these two databases to look at the predicted value of antibiotic treatment. The only problems we face with this are legal ones.

Lipsitch: How did the actual numbers of resistant cases change after the prescribing behaviour changed? Did the number of resistant isolates go down or simply the percentage as a fraction of all isolates?

Huovinen: I assume that the number of samples we have received has been quite stable, with no large differences between 1991 and 1995. Thus the fraction of resistant isolates will have decreased.

Reference

Levin BR, Lipsitch M, Perrot V et al 1997 The population genetics of antibiotic resistance. Clin Infect Dis, in press

The contribution of antibiotic use on the frequency of antibiotic resistance in hospitals

Robert Gaynes and Dominique Monnet

Hospital Infections Program, MS E-55, Centers for Disease Control and Prevention, 1600 Clifton Road, Atlanta, GA 30333, USA and C.CLIN, Sud-Est, Centre Hospitalier Lyon-Sud, Pavillon 1M, Pierre-Benite Cedex, 69495, France

Abstract. Abundant evidence suggests a relationship between antibiotic resistance and use, including animal models, consistent associations between resistance and antibiotic use in hospitals, concomitant variation in resistance as antibiotic use varies, and a dose–response relationship for many pathogen/antibiotic combinations. Much of the evidence has come from studies performed in single hospitals. Most multicentre studies on resistance have not included data on antibiotic usage. Despite this substantial body of evidence, some studies have failed to demonstrate an association between antibiotic resistance and use, suggesting other contributing factors such as cross-transmission, inter-hospital transfer of resistance, a community contribution to resistance, or a complex relationship between resistance and the use of a variety of antibiotics. A multicentre study, project ICARE (Intensive Care Antimicrobial Resistance Epidemiology), implemented in 1994 by Centers for Disease Control and Prevention and Rollins School of Public Health, Emory University, has found dramatic differences in the patterns of antibiotic usage and resistance in US hospitals. The findings suggest that antibiotic usage is the major risk factor in development of antibiotic resistance in hospitals but the relationship can be complex with additional factors involved. Understanding the problem of antibiotic resistance in a hospital cannot be achieved without knowledge of the hospital's pattern of antibiotic use.

1997 Antibiotic resistance: origins, evolution, selection and spread. Wiley, Chichester (Ciba Foundation Symposium 207) p 47–60

Perhaps no other class of pharmaceutical agents has had such a major impact on public health as antibiotics. Early in this century infectious diseases were among the most common causes of death. Largely because of antibiotics, these same diseases all but disappeared from the causes of death in the US population. Unfortunately, some of these same diseases are reappearing, this time largely due to the failure of antibiotics. For the first time since their introduction, we are faced with the loss of efficacy of antibiotics. Multidrug-resistant tuberculosis and vancomycin-resistant enterococci are often untreatable.

The relationship between antibiotic use and antibiotic resistance seems obvious at first glance. However, the relationship is often more complex, since some studies do not show a clear relationship between antibiotic use and resistance. The objective of this paper is to examine this relationship and determine alternative explanations for antibiotic resistance in hospitals when antibiotic use fails to explain it.

The relationship between antibiotic resistance and antibiotic use from a biological model

A clear relationship between antibiotic use and resistance has been shown by a biological model. Developed by Levy et al (1976), this animal model for selection and dissemination of tetracycline-resistant *Escherichia coli* in chickens receiving oxytetracycline-supplemented feed showed a strong relationship between the introduction of the antibiotic and development of resistance. Antibiotic resistance among pathogens isolated from humans quickly followed the clinical introduction of many antibiotics (US Congress 1995, CDC 1994, Coronado et al 1995).

The unique nature of the hospital environment

Whereas a relationship may exist between antibiotic use and antibiotic resistance in any environment, the hospital environment is uniquely suited to such a relationship. Most (Bryce & Smith 1995, Yu et al 1979, Gaynes 1995) but not all (McGowan et al 1989) studies suggest that resistance is greater among pathogens isolated from hospitalized patients than among those isolated from patients in the community. In a multicentre study, project ICARE (Intensive Care Antimicrobial Resistance Epidemiology), implemented in 1994 by Centers for Disease Control and Prevention and Rollins School of Public Health, Emory University, information was collected from the microbiology laboratories of eight US hospitals (Monnet et al 1995). These hospitals reported nosocomial infections, pathogens and susceptibilities from the intensive care unit (ICU) surveillance component in the National Nosocomial Infections Surveillance (NNIS) system (Emori et al 1991). For project ICARE they provided additional data from the microbiology laboratory and pharmacy. The data for certain antibiotic/pathogen combinations were stratified for each ICU, for the non-ICU inpatient wards combined, and for outpatients, e.g. the percentage of methicillin-resistant *Staphylococcus aureus* (MRSA) from these wards. Data from this pilot study showed that for eight out of ten pathogen/antibiotic combinations examined, the percentage resistant was higher in the hospital than in the outpatient isolates. More specifically, the percentage resistant was higher in the isolates from the ICUs than from the other inpatient areas (Fig. 1).

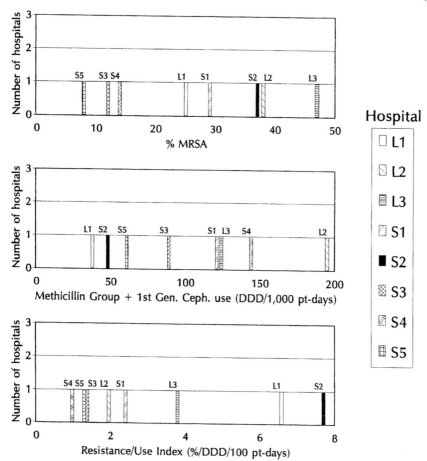

FIG. 1. Distribution of hospitals by percentage of methicillin-, nafcillin-, or oxacillin-resistant *Staphylococcus aureus* (MRSA). Hospitals are denoted by L1–L3 (>500 beds) or S1–S5 (<500 beds). The percentage of all *S. aureus* that were MRSA can be seen in the top graph. The antibiotic use data can be seen for the same hospitals in the middle graph as expressed as defined daily doses (DDD)/1000 patient days. To control for the effect of antibiotic use, we calculated a resistance/use index, seen on the bottom graph, by dividing the percentage MRSA by the antibiotic use expressed as DDD/100 patient days. Outpatient data for the hospitals were excluded in all graphs. Ceph., cephalosporin. Source: NNIS/ICARE.

The importance of the intensive care unit

The higher percentage resistant in the isolates from the ICUs is reflected in many studies (Bryce & Smith 1995, Yu et al 1979, Gaynes 1995, Flaherty & Weinstein 1996). For example, in the NNIS System, over 230 participating hospitals voluntarily send data on nosocomial infections, their associated pathogens, and the pathogens' susceptibility profiles to Centers for Disease Control and Prevention. These pathogens represent a subset of those isolated from a ward or unit in the hospital since they must be associated with a nosocomial infection (Emori et al 1991). On the basis of NNIS data, resistance to vancomycin is increasing among *Enterococcus* spp., especially from isolates associated with nosocomial infections in ICUs. Most of these vancomycin-resistant enterococci (VRE) are resistant to all currently available antibiotics (Frieden et al 1993, Centers for Disease Control 1993). As a consequence, treatment options for patients with nosocomial infections associated with VRE are limited often to unproven combinations of antibiotics or experimental compounds. Among certain Gram-negative bacilli resistance is also increasing. From NNIS data, the percentage of *Klebsiella pneumoniae* isolates resistant to extended-spectrum β-lactams increased from 0.5% in 1986 to 12% in 1993 (Monnet et al 1994). NNIS data also suggested inter-hospital spread of resistant *K. pneumoniae* in the geographical region surrounding one NNIS hospital, where the pathogen spread from one of the NNIS hospital's ICU. Reports from the NNIS system parallel others highlighting the role of the ICU in the development of increasing resistance among nosocomial isolates of *S. aureus*, *Enterococcus* spp., *Enterobacter* spp. and *Pseudomonas aeruginosa* (Voss et al 1994, Panlilio et al 1992, Bryce & Smith 1995, Gaynes & Culver 1992, Burwen et al 1994, McGowan et al 1989).

The reasons for the unique nature of the hospital environment are varied. Factors that might increase the risk for antibiotic resistance in a hospital, and ICUs in particular, include cross-transmission of pathogens between closely quartered patients, lack of asepsis during crisis care, transfer of patients colonized with resistant pathogens between units or other hospitals, or introduction of resistant organisms from the community by patients or healthcare workers. The latter is particularly a problem when nursing home patients are continually transferred to area hospitals.

Prevalence of antibiotic use in hospitals

Perhaps no other factor is more important in the development of antibiotic resistance than antibiotic use in hospitals. Approximately 25–40% of all hospitalized patients receive antibiotics (Cooke et al 1980, Scheckler & Bennett 1970, Kunin et al 1973, McGowan & Finland 1979, Shapiro et al 1979, Chow et al 1991, Evans & Kortas 1996). Many antibiotics are used only or primarily in hospitals. Doses of antibiotics are often higher in hospitals, especially with parenteral administration. This higher dosing creates a strong selective pressure for resistance.

Consistent association between antibiotic resistance and antibiotic use in hospitals

Several studies in hospitals have examined the relationship between antibiotic resistance and antibiotic use. Of such studies, 22 reviewed by McGowan (1983) have shown a fairly consistent association. Importantly, most of the studies have shown a dose–response relationship that is usually linear (Pallares et al 1993, Søgaard 1989). Unfortunately, nearly all of these studies were reports from single hospitals, which may represent a bias and not necessarily the situation in other hospitals. Few multicentre studies have examined this relationship. Among these are studies performed in several hospitals in the 1970s in the United States that examined aminoglycoside use and aminoglycoside resistance among Gram-negative bacilli (Gerding & Larson 1986, Muscato et al 1991), a study by the National Nosocomial Resistance Surveillance Group in the 1980s (Ballow & Schentag 1992) and, in the 1990s, project ICARE (Monnet et al 1995). Project ICARE collects data from its participating hospitals on antibiotic use. The antibiotic use data (expressed as defined daily dose of antibiotic/1000 patient days) are reported for each ICU and for non-ICU inpatient wards combined. However, in this project, information on antibiotic use outside the hospital is not accessible for collection. Results from these studies shed some light on the nature of the relationship between antibiotic resistance and use.

Concomitant variation in antibiotic use leading to changes in antibiotic resistance

Most but not all hospitals involved in the collection of the aminoglycoside resistance/ use data collection found that changes in antibiotic use led to parallel changes in resistance. The National Nosocomial Resistance Surveillance Group found similar variations but also found that the relationship was not necessarily maintained for all antibiotic/pathogen combinations. For example, for ceftazidime use a linear relationship was apparent for ceftazidime-resistant *Enterobacter cloacae* but not for ceftazidime-resistant *P. aeruginosa*.

The complex relationship between antibiotic resistance and antibiotic use in hospitals

The complexity of this relationship was also evident in the pilot phase of Project ICARE which examined the percentage of MRSA (Fig. 1, top graph) and antibiotic use data for the same hospitals (Fig. 1, middle graph). For two hospitals with nearly identical percentages of MRSA (Hospitals S1 and L2), the combined antibiotic use data for methicillin, oxacillin, nafcillin, dicloxacillin, cloxacillin and first-generation cephalosporins differ dramatically.

To control for the effect of antibiotic use, we calculated a resistance/use index (Fig. 1, bottom graph). If a hospital has a high resistance/use index, this may indicate that the percentage resistant is due to some aspect other than antibiotic selective pressure, e.g. cross-transmission or resistance from the community.

Although data from project ICARE help a hospital determine whether its antimicrobial usage is, in part, responsible for antibiotic resistance, confounding variables such as variation in case mix, e.g. transplant patients requiring multiple

TABLE 1   Distribution of hospitals' use of selected classes of antibiotics

Hospital[a]	Antibiotic class				
	Anti-staphylococcal penicillins and first-generation cephalosporins	Vancomycin	Ceftazidime	Third-generation cephalosporins	Fluoroquinolones
L1	38	16	13	17	21
L2	195	70	103	154	74
L3	124	52	19	135	17
S1	121	30	40	75	45
S2	48	10	25	94	54
S3	89	12	32	98	50
S4	144	28	20	78	41
S5	61	18	10	41	23

Figures given represent defined daily dosages per 1000 patient days.
Source: Phase I of Project ICARE (see text for details).
[a]L1, L2, L3 refer to hospitals ≥ 500 beds; S1–S5 refer to hospitals < 500 beds.

antimicrobial agents might account for disparate hospital antimicrobial use that may be unrelated to selective pressure for resistance.

Are hospitals optimizing their use of antibiotics?

There were striking differences between project ICARE hospitals in the amounts of antibiotics used. Table 1 shows the use of the anti-staphylococcal penicillins, first-generation cephalosporins, vancomycin, ceftazidime, third-generation cephalosporins and fluoroquinolones by size of hospital from phase I of project ICARE. The results are very limited due to the small numbers of hospitals in phase I; none the less, one hospital, L2, ranked highest in using each class of antibiotic which has prompted close examination of prescribing strategy in that hospital.

Examining antibiotic use in a hospital

Once an institution determines whether or not it is overusing antibiotics with comparative data such as those provided by project ICARE, close examination of the patterns of antibiotic use is needed. Studies suggest that antibiotic use can be divided into three categories: empirical therapy, definitive therapy and prophylaxis. Surprisingly, only about 30% of all antibiotics in hospitals are used for definitive therapy where the susceptibility patterns for the infection-associated pathogen are

TABLE 2 Strategies available for changing prescribing practices

---

Educational and persuasive strategies
Educational conferences
Feedback of prescribing data
Guidelines (requires feedback loop)

Facilitative strategies
Clinical specialist (e.g. pharmacist) consultation
Computer help screens when ordering antibiotics

Power strategies
Control of contact between pharmaceutical representatives and prescribers
Formularies
Restriction of use by requiring approval
Automatic stop orders

---

known (Scheckler & Bennett 1970, Kunin et al 1973). About one third of all antibiotics are used for prophylaxis. Inappropriate use such as unnecessary therapy, poor drug choice, misguided prophylaxis, or inappropriate dosing occurred in 41% of cases in one hospital, underscoring the need for more effective programs examining antibiotic use (Cooke et al 1980, Maki & Schuna 1978).

A variety of approaches have been advocated to optimize antibiotic use in hospitals ranging from formulary restrictions to pharmacist intervention (Table 2) (Avorn et al 1987). These approaches have usually been effective in reducing inappropriate use, but their effectiveness in reducing antibiotic resistance in the hospital has been difficult to assess. Some studies showed a decrease in resistance with restrictive use of aminoglycosides such as gentamicin and tobramycin (Gerding & Larson 1986, Muscato et al 1991), but these restrictions were offset by increases in amikacin use and, in some instances, increased amikacin resistance.

To assist hospital leaders in reducing antimicrobial resistance, a multidisciplinary group of experts has developed five strategic goals to optimize antibiotic use: (1) optimizing antibiotic prophylaxis for operative procedures; (2) optimizing choice and duration of empirical therapy; (3) improving antibiotic prescribing practice by educational and administrative means; (4) monitoring and providing feedback regarding antibiotic resistance within a hospital; and (5) defining and implementing healthcare delivery system guidelines for important types of antibiotic use (Goldmann et al 1996). Each of these goals has suggested measurements for gauging progress that would allow institutions to improve their antibiotic use.

A challenge to hospital leadership

No strategy for controlling antibiotic resistance or optimizing antibiotic use will be successful unless the entire healthcare delivery system views these problems as vital ones. We can no longer rely on pharmaceutical companies to bail us out of this predicament — drug companies cannot guarantee they will find a new class of antibiotics. Since the introduction of quinolones in the 1980s, no new class of antibiotics has been introduced. Recent reports have shown that resistance to this class of drugs occurred with alarming swiftness (Coronado et al 1995). The solution to the problem of antibiotic resistance in hospitals cannot be solved solely by the repetitive introduction of new antibiotics. It will be too costly and it will be a strategy that will ultimately fail. Witness the problems with vancomycin-resistant enterococci.

Physicians and infection control practitioners do not preside over the complex interdepartmental and multidisciplinary systems that influence the introduction, dissemination and control of antibiotic use and resistance. Success depends on the hospital leadership developing programs to improve these serious problems. These programs must, however, be grounded in sound data collection, analysis, and interpretation.

Conclusions

Several considerations must be kept in mind when evaluating antimicrobial resistance and usage in hospitals. Interpretation of the magnitude of antibiotic resistance in hospitals cannot be made without knowledge of a hospital's pattern of antibiotic use. Since the ICU is often the focus of resistance in a hospital, the ICU and non-ICU inpatient areas should be examined separately. Dramatic differences exist in patterns of antibiotic resistance and use in hospitals. In particular, a high prevalence of resistance did not necessarily correlate with heavy antibiotic use. By improving our monitoring, we can determine the relative need of hospitals to focus on antimicrobial use and its control, or on other efforts such as prevention of cross-infection caused by resistant pathogens. Because of the dramatic increases in antimicrobial resistance in hospitals, truly effective control measures are needed including examination of antibiotic use and infection control practices.

References

Avorn J, Harvey K, Soumerai S et al 1987 Information and education as determinants of antibiotic use: report of Task Force 5. Rev Infect Dis 9:286S–296S

Ballow CH, Schentag JJ 1992 Trends in antibiotic utilization and bacterial resistance: report of the National Nosocomial Resistance Surveillance Group. Diagn Microbiol Infect Dis 15:37S–42S

Bryce EA, Smith JA 1995 Focused microbiological surveillance and Gram-negative β-lactamase mediated resistance in an intensive care unit. Infect Control Hosp Epidemiol 16:331–334

Burwen DR, Banerjee SN, Gaynes RP 1994 Ceftazidime resistance among selected nosocomial Gram-negative bacilli in the United States. J Infect Dis 170:1622–1625

Centers for Disease Control 1993 Nosocomial enterococci resistant to vancomycin: United States 1989–1993. Morb Mortal Wkly Rep 42:597–599

Centers for Disease Control 1994 Addressing emerging infectious disease threats: a prevention strategy for the United States. US Department of Health and Human Services, Atlanta, GA

Chow JW, Fine MJ, Shlaes DM et al 1991 *Enterobacter* bacteremia: clinical features and emergence of antibiotic resistance during therapy. Ann Intern Med 115:585–590

Cooke DM, Salter AJ, Phillips I 1980 Antimicrobial misuse, antibiotic policies and information resources. J Antimicrob Chemother 6:435–443

Coronado VG, Edwards JR, Culver DH, Gaynes RP 1995 Ciprofloxacin resistance among nosocomial *Pseudomonas aeruginosa* and *Staphylococcus aureus* in the United States. Infect Control Hosp Epidemiol 16:71–75

Emori TG, Culver DH, Horan TC et al 1991 The National Nosocomial Infections Surveillance (NNIS) System: description of surveillance methods. Am J Infect Control 19:19–35

Evans ME, Kortas KJ 1996 Vancomycin use in a university medical center: comparison with Hospital Infection Control Practices Advisory Committee guidelines. Infect Control Hosp Epidemiol 17:356–359

Flaherty JP, Weinstein RA 1996 Nosocomial infections caused by antibiotic-resistant organisms in the intensive care unit. Infect Control Hosp Epidemiol 17:236–248

Frieden TR, Munsiff SS, Low DE et al 1993 Emergence of vancomycin-resistant *Enterococcus* in New York City. Lancet 342:490–491

Gaynes R 1995 Antibiotic resistance in ICUs: a multifaceted problem requiring a multifaceted solution. Infect Control Hosp Epidemiol 16:328–330

Gaynes RP, Culver DH 1992 The National Nosocomial Infections Surveillance System. Resistance to imipenem among selected Gram-negative bacilli in the United States. Infect Control Hosp Epidemiol 13:10–14

Gerding DN, Larson TA 1986 Resistance surveillance programs and the incidence of Gram-negative bacillary resistance to amikacin from 1967–1985. Am J Med 80:22–28

Goldmann DA, Weinstein RA, Wenzel R et al 1996 Strategies to prevent and control the emergence and spread of antimicrobial-resistant microorganisms in hospitals. A challenge to hospital leadership. JAMA 275:234–240

Kunin CM, Tupasi T, Craig WA 1973 Use of antibiotics. A brief exposition of the problem and some tentative solutions. Ann Intern Med 79:555–560

Levy SB, Fitzgerald GG, Macone AB 1976 Changes in intestinal flora of farm personnel after introduction of tetracycline-supplemented feed on a farm. N Engl J Med 295:583–588

Maki DG, Schuna AA 1978 A study of antimicrobial misuse in a university hospital. Am J Med Sci 275:271–282

McGowan JE 1983 Antimicrobial resistance in hospital organisms and its relation to antibiotic use. Rev Infect Dis 5:1033–1048

McGowan JE, Finland M 1974 Infection and antibiotic use at Boston City Hospital: changes in prevalence during the decade. J Infect Dis 129:421–428

McGowan JE Jr, Hall EC, Parrott PL 1989 Antimicrobial susceptibility in Gram-negative bacteremia: are nosocomial isolates really more resistant? Antimicrob Agents Chemother 33:1855–1859

Monnet D, Edwards J, Gaynes R 1994 The National Nosocomial Infections Surveillance (NNIS) System. Extended spectrum β-lactam-resistant nosocomial *Klebsiella pneumoniae* (ESB-KP): epidemiologic evidence of interhospital transmission. Infect Control Hosp Epidemiol (suppl) 15:23

Monnet D, Gaynes R, Tenover F, McGowan J 1995 Ceftazidime-resistant *Pseudomonas aeruginosa* and ceftazidime usage in NNIS hospitals: preliminary results of Project ICARE, Phase one. Infect Control Hosp Epidemiol (suppl) 4:19

Muscato JJ, Wilbur DW, Stout JJ, Fahrlender RA 1991 An evaluation of the susceptibility patterns of gram-negative organisms isolated in cancer centers with aminoglycoside usage. J Antimicrob Chemother (suppl C) 27:1–7

Pallares R, Dick R, Wenzel R, Adams JR, Nettleman MD 1993 Trends in antimicrobial utilization at a tertiary teaching hospital during a 15-year period (1978–1992). Infect Control Hosp Epidemiol 14:376–382

Panlilio AL, Culver DH, Gaynes RP et al 1992 Methicillin-resistant *Staphylococcus aureus* in US hospitals, 1975–1991. Infect Control Hosp Epidemiol 13:582–586

Scheckler WE, Bennett JV 1970 Antibiotic use in seven community hospitals. JAMA 213:264–267

Shapiro M, Townsend TR, Rosner B, Kass EH 1979 Use of antimicrobial drugs in general hospitals. II: Analysis of patterns of use. J Infect Dis 139:698–706

Søgaard P 1989 The epidemiology of antibiotic resistance in three species of the *Enterobacteriaceae* and the relation to consumption of antimicrobial agents in Odense University Hospital. Dan Med Bull 36:65–84

US Congress 1995 Office of Technology Assessment. Impacts of antibiotic-resistant bacteria, OTA-H-629. US Government Printing Office, Washington, DC

Voss A, Milatovic D, Wallrauch-Schwartz C, Rosdahl VT, Braveny I 1994 Methicillin-resistant *Staphylococcus aureus* in Europe. Eur J Clin Microbiol Infect Dis 13:50–55

Yu VL, Oakes CA, Axnick KJ, Merigan TC 1979 Patient factors contributing to the emergence of gentamicin-resistant *Serratia marcescens*. Am J Med 44:468–473

DISCUSSION

Lerner: In the hospital setting, patients with organisms such as VRE that are no longer treatable with available drugs have caught the eye of the surgeons. Consequently, for the first time, surgeons now are willing to consider modifying their profligate prophylactic use of vancomycin.

You make a distinction between ICU use and ward use. Much of antimicrobial therapy, including parenteral therapy, has begun to move out of the hospital—either we push patients to oral therapy or continue parenteral therapy outside the hospital. What do you expect to be the consequences of this?

Gaynes: There have been many issues in the USA in particular about home health care, not the least of which has been the fact that we have recently investigated four epidemics of bloodstream infections with unusual resistance, that have been related to home health care agencies. Getting the data is a remarkable problem because when home health care agencies have a problem that requires a patient to go back into the hospital it is very difficult to get the two to talk to each other. The patient is diagnosed with the infection in the hospital but the home health care agency doesn't know anything about it, because all they've done is transfer the patient. In terms of my speculation as to what's going to happen, because of the fact that you are effectively isolating the patient by sending them home, the chances of resistance due to cross-transmission are greatly diminished. But if I'm correct in assuming that the dominant risk factor for resistance in a hospital is antibiotic exposure, resistance will continue to be a problem albeit at a slightly reduced level.

Davies: If you compare hospital L1 with hospital L2, is there any difference in morbidity and mortality between the two?

Gaynes: In this system I have to be very careful about protecting the confidentiality of the hospitals: if I start releasing their names, many of which you would recognize immediately, I would stop getting data. The answer to your question is that there is probably no difference. However, when you look at every single class of antibiotics, hospital L2 is by far the highest user. They had to look very seriously at their prescribing practices, which they are now doing.

Sköld: We did a survey of the nine largest Swedish hospitals regarding the use of antibiotics (measured as defined daily doses per 1000 patient days). We found dramatic differences between them, despite the fact that the patient groups are homogenous and the panorama of infections is similar. For example, one hospital used six times as much tetracycline as another. Penicillins normally constitute more than half of the antibiotics used and cephalosporins about 15%, but one hospital used 40% cephalosporins and just about 30% penicillins. These are inexplicable differences.

Levy: Did you ever find out why?

Sköld: I tried hard to interest the social medicine people in following this up, but no one wanted to do it.

Levy: Yours is the only study of which I'm aware that has clearly demonstrated enormous differences in antibiotic prescribing in hospitals of similar size in a country with a rather homogeneous population.

Gaynes: We've expanded what I've shown you today: we now have almost 50 hospitals collecting similar data. We intend to identify more hospitals like L2 that appear to be high antibiotic users and others that are not in an effort to determine reasons for the rather remarkable diversity that I showed you from just eight. We want to go into these hospitals and look at the highs and the lows to identify the differences in prescribing practices. I think this is an essential issue.

Cohen: It is difficult to predict the impact of prescribing practices on infection and resistance, because physicians are often using antibiotics on the basis of pharmacodynamics rather than susceptibility. For example, for penicillin-susceptible infections, physicians are using extended-spectrum cephalosporins that can be given once a day to treat people as outpatients, rather than using penicillin which must be given four or five times a day in the hospital. It's hard to predict the consequences of such practices. We may start seeing VRE as a community-acquired problem.

Gaynes: I wouldn't be surprised. It's already changing in our database as well.

Bush: Some hospitals are trying to cycle antibiotics. Do you think this will change the profile of resistance?

Gaynes: We had a meeting recently to look at phase III issues, and this was one that was discussed. If you look at the literature on cycling of antibiotics (John McGowan [1994] has done to my knowledge the only review of this), there's no agreement on how to cycle, how long to cycle for and what to use. Most of the studies are equivocal in answering the question as to whether this strategy will work. Yet, when we talk to various people that are involved in our project, there's tremendous interest in it.

Witte: Multicentre studies performed in Germany from 1990, by the end of 1995 had shown that intensive care units are more often affected by multiresistant organisms than other units. It could be shown by molecular typing that not only do they spread within particular hospitals but also that there is dissemination between hospitals.

Gaynes: Do you get a feel for how much cross-transmission is occurring in terms of resistance compared with selective pressure from antibiotics?

Witte: That is hard to assess. A student in our laboratory has now looked at three district hospitals with sporadic staphylococcal infections. By typing isolates we have looked at how often cross-transmission might have occurred in endemic situations. It is less than 5% (K. Reiber & W. Witte, unpublished results).

Summers: Going back to Bruce Levin's population issues, it's easy to get resistances to go up and hard to get them to come back down for reasons we don't completely understand. Is the correlation of use and resistance only examined on the upswing, where if more is being used we can see resistance go up, or are there occasions where follow-on studies have been done to quantify the decline in resistance? All of these steady-states really depend on the decay rate.

Gaynes: There are only a few studies that show that if you decrease antibiotic use, you decrease resistance; the only multicentre study was the one that I mentioned where if aminoglycoside (gentamicin) use was decreased, resistance was clearly decreased. Many people have looked at ways of decreasing antibiotic use but, amazingly, they didn't look at resistance.

Giamarellou: Is there any evidence from the literature regarding multiresistant Gram-negatives proving that even if the correct antibiotic is administered (according to the susceptibility pattern) these multiresistant strains might be more virulent? Genes for resistance are often plasmid-borne: might there also be genes for virulence on the same plasmid?

Gaynes: I don't know the answer to that question. One parallel study in hospital infections looked at VRE infections compared with VSE, and showed that if you had VRE in your bloodstream you were more likely to die, suggesting increased virulence (Shay et al 1995). A study we did on this failed to show a significant difference (Stroud et al 1996). Other than these, it has been difficult to look at that question.

Piddock: When we studied ceftazidime resistance, we found it very difficult to transfer the ESBL (extended spectrum β-lactamase) plasmid if we used ceftazidime as a selector: we found it much easier if we used other antibiotic resistances (e.g. ampicillin) on that plasmid (Piddock et al 1996). As ICUs are notorious for using multiple antibiotic regimens, I wonder whether it might not be the ceftazidime consumption that is influencing the level of ceftazidime resistance, but rather the use of something else selecting the plasmid. This might explain why your two hospitals aren't influenced by the ceftazidime consumption. If you were to look at, for instance, gentamicin, this might be what is causing your similar levels of resistance.

Bush: There are at least two instances in the literature where ceftazidime use has been decreased and the number of ceftazidime-resistant strains of *Klebsiella* have decreased in a hospital (Meyer et al 1993, Naumovski et al 1992).

Lipsitch: In hospitals where you had a strong correlation in the ICU but no correlation outside, it would be interesting to see what would happen if you plotted antibiotic use in the ICU on the X-axis and resistance outside the ICU on the Y-axis.

Gaynes: We've looked at that but we have not been able to show any correlation: I was surprised that we didn't find much.

One of the reasons that we haven't shown a relationship in the in-patient area as well as we have in the ICU could be that we may have over-lumped the in-patient areas. There are quite a variety of approaches for examining antibiotics and resistance in various areas in the hospital. For instance, there may be major differences between a cancer ward compared with an ophthalmology ward. We may have over-lumped that for the sake of ease of data collection.

Summers: In the context of this discipline, is it not the case that a 50% correct guess constitutes certainty?

Gaynes: There are only about half a dozen studies in the literature that fail to show that the relationship between use and resistance, and at least the 22 plus the various multicentre studies that I've described have shown that there is a very strong relationship. There's overwhelming evidence in my view that the two are related. I'm trying to show that the relationship seems the strongest from what we can see preliminarily in the ICU.

Baquero: All these studies should be complemented by cross-transmission studies. Differences between hospitals may be entirely due to epidemics — either epidemics of resistant organisms or epidemics of susceptible organisms which are hitting the possibility of looking at resistant ones.

Gaynes: We are looking at that. The first step was confirming the susceptibility patterns of what the hospitals sent us, which we have done virtually in all cases. We have looked for epidemics and actually not found very much.

Baquero: What is the relationship between the ability of a strain to cause epidemics and antibiotic resistance?

Gaynes: Epidemics with resistant strains are investigated rather thoroughly because the resistance markers are so obvious in a hospital. A large percentage of the time in those epidemics antibiotic use also comes up as an important risk factor even when strain typing suggests cross-transmission of the resistant organisms.

Huovinen: If you decrease consumption of ceftazidime, the problem is that is replaced by other antimicrobial agents.

Gaynes: That's the part we don't know about. It's amazing to me in the literature how often a total reduction in overall use of antibiotic is shown without anyone reporting the resistance change.

Levy: In summarizing, there are differences between a closed ICU containing 5–10 patients who are somewhat isolated and the rest of the hospital, where patients are more moveable and there is more change in patient stay and medication. In the whole hospital there are many other variables which complicate looking at change by examining one variable, the antibiotic. It is of interest, however, that Pentti Huovinen could discuss reduced use of erythromycin and decrease of resistance in a large area, where these people are mixing with the general population. In the hospitals it's a different situation since patients are coming in and out and the location is more confined.

References

McGowan JE Jr 1994 Do intensive hospital antibiotic control programs prevent the spread of antibiotic resistance? Infect Control Hosp Epidemiol 17:478–483

Meyer KS, Urban C, Eagan JA, Berger BJ, Rahal JJ 1993 Nosocomial outbreak of *Klebsiella* infection resistant to late generation cephalosporins. Ann Intern Med 119:353–358

Naumovski L, Quinn JP, Miyashiro D et al 1992 Outbreak of ceftazidime resistance due to a novel extended spectrum β-lactamase in isolates from cancer patients. Antimicrob Agents Chemother 36:1991–1996

Piddock LJV, Walters RN, Jin Y-F, Turner HL, Gascoyne-Binzi DM, Hawkey PM 1996 Prevalence and mechanism of resistance to 'third generation' cephalosporins in clinically relevant isolates of Enterobacteriaceae from 43 hospitals in the United Kingdom between May 1990 and May 1991. J Antimicrob Chemother, in press

Shay DK, Maloney SA, Montecalvo M et al 1995 Epidemiology and mortality risk of vancomycin-resistant enterococci bloodstream infections. J Infect Dis 172:993–1000

Stroud L, Edwards J, Danzig L, Culver D, Gaynes R 1996 Risk factors for mortality associated with enterococcal bloodstream infections. Infect Control Hosp Epidemiol 17:576–580

Impact of antibiotic use in animal feeding on resistance of bacterial pathogens in humans

Wolfgang Witte

Robert Koch-Institute, Wernigerode Branch, Burgstraße 37, D-38855 Wernigerode, Germany

Abstract. With the exception of flavomycin and olaquindox, the antibiotics currently used in European countries as feed additives exert a Gram-positive spectrum of activity. Of these, tylosin and virginiamycin are known for cross-resistance to macrolides, lincosamidines and streptogramines, and avoparcin is known for cross-resistance to vancomycin and teicoplanin. The use of avoparcin in animal husbandry creates a potential reservoir of transferable, *vanA*-mediated glycopeptide resistance in enterococci. A study in a rural area in Germany where vancomycin-resistant enterococci (VRE) were not isolated from infected humans but found in animal husbandry has shown that VRE are disseminated via meat products and are also found in faecal samples of non-hospitalized humans. VRE of different ecological origin from Germany (hospitals, sewage, food, animal husbandry) are polyclonal as evidenced by macrorestriction patterns and multilocus enzyme electrophoresis, suggesting a wide dissemination of the *vanA* gene cluster. These results confirm earlier observations on the spread of the *sat* genes, which confer resistance to a streptothricin antibiotic which has only been used in animal feeding. The resistance determinants were later also found in *Escherichia coli* from human infections and had spread in the absence of selective pressure.

1997 Antibiotic resistance: origins, evolution, selection and spread. Wiley, Chichester (Ciba Foundation Symposium 207) p 61–75

Antibiotics have been used as growth promoters in animal feeding for several decades. Soon after the detection of transferable antibiotic resistance in Enterobacteriaceae, animal production was identified as a potential reservoir of resistance determinants. At that time, oxytetracycline was the main antibiotic used as feed additive, and a number of investigations showed a strong association between ergotropic tetracycline use and the frequency of tetracycline resistance in enterobacterial isolates from animals and livestock workers (Levy et al 1976a,b). As a consequence, at least in the European Community (EC), further use of tetracycline for this purpose was prohibited. The World Health Organization (WHO) recommended that antibiotics which select for resistance against antibiotics used for human chemotherapy should no longer be used in animal husbandry, a demand renewed in 1994 (WHO 1995). In the 1980s, relevant EC authorities established legislation for the use of antibacterial agents as growth promoters in animal husbandry, prohibiting the use of substances selecting for resistance to antibacterial agents used in human chemotherapy (Helmuth & Bulling 1985).

Although new candidate antibacterial growth promoters must fulfil this criterion for them to be passed by regulatory boards, there are a number of antibiotics that have been used as growth promoters for more than 20 years for which cross-resistance to antibiotics used in human chemotherapy is known (Table 1). A fresh evaluation of these substances in the light of the recent development of drug resistance in Gram-positive pathogens seems to be necessary.

Looking at the ergotropic use of these antibiotics as one of the possible sources for emergence and spread of transferable resistance, the following questions have to be answered:

(1) Does ergotropic use of antibiotics really select for resistance?
(2) Is cross-resistance to antibiotics used in human chemotherapy determined by the same resistance mechanism in strains from both animal and human sources?
(3) Are the corresponding resistance determinants disseminated via the food chain, and to what extent are they found in the intestinal flora of non-hospitalized humans?

In connection with the increasing clinical significance of vancomycin resistance in enterococci (Frieden et al 1993) it is of great interest to answer these questions with regard to the ergotropic use of avoparcin.

Glycopeptide resistance in enterococci

Resistance to glycopeptides is more often found in *Enterococcus faecium* than in *E. faecalis*. Although glycopeptide resistance was found in 8% of enterococci from nosocomial infections in the United States in 1993 (Centers for Disease Control 1993), it was rarer (0.7–1%) among clinical isolates in Central Europe at the beginning of the 1990s but reached 5% in *E. faecium* at the end of 1995 (M. Kresken, personal communication).

Most glycopeptide-resistant enterococci possess the inducible high level type resistance that is encoded by the *vanA* gene cluster, carried on transposons similar or related to Tn*1546*. It can be easily transferred if it is located on conjugative plasmids. The main constituent of the resistance mechanism is the VanA protein, a ligase of broad substrate specificity. It is responsible for the synthesis of depsipeptides, which can be incorporated into peptidoglyccan precursors instead of the D-alanine dipeptide (Courvalin 1990). Obviously, less frequent in enterococci is the *vanB* type of resistance, which is inducible by vancomycin but not by teicoplanin (Evers et al 1993). The constitutive chromosome-encoded low level resistance $vanC_1$ phenotype is likely a species characteristic of *E. gallinarum*, as is the $vanC_2$ phenotype for *E. casseliflavus* (Navarro & Courvalin 1994).

TABLE 1 Antibacterial substances used as feed additives in animal husbandry in European countries

Compound	Class	Mode of action	Known resistance mechanisms	Cross-resistance
Olaquindox	Quinoxaline	Inhibition of DNA synthesis	NO reduction	Other quinoxalines
Zn-Bacitracin	Polypeptide	Inhibits dephosphorylation of undecaprenyl pyrophosphate lipid carrier of cell wall precursors	Spontaneous mutants not characterized	Unknown
Flavomycin	Phosphoglycolipid	Inhibition of cell wall synthesis	Unknown	Unknown
Monensin, salinomycin	Ionophore	Disaggregation of cytoplasmic membrane	Unknown	Unknown
Tylosin	Macrolide	Binding to the 50S ribosomal subunit inhibition of binding aminoacyl-tRNAs and of peptidyl transferase	Methylation of 23S rRNA in position 2058	When constitutive; all macrolides, lincosamidines, streptogramin-β-antibiotics
Virginiamycin	Streptogramin	Inhibition of conformational change of the 24S ribosomal protein, preventing protein chain extension	O-hydrolase, porter mechanism	Other streptogramin antibiotics
Avoparcin	Glycopeptide	Inhibition of transglycosylation	Modification of the peptidoglycan precursor	Vancoycmin, teicoplanin, daptomycin, avoparcin

Shortly after the first report of the natural occurrence of vancomycin-resistant *E. faecium* (VRE) possessing the *vanA*-mediated resistance mechanism, numerous outbreaks of VRE had been recorded in the USA (Centers for Disease Control 1995). Although not all of the VRE isolates from these outbreaks were subjected to molecular typing, there are examples for both exogenous infections by spread of a particular strain, presumably related to poor hospital hygiene, and endogenous infections as indicated by different typing patterns of corresponding enterococcal isolates (Bingen et al 1991). The latter finding suggests that VRE has spread among the community and may have become part of the intestinal flora of patients entering hospitals. The widespread presence of VRE outside hospitals had already been established by isolation from sewage treatment plants (Klare et al 1993, Torres et al 1994).

The discovery of VRE in a sewage treatment plant in a rural area of former East Germany with no or only exceptional and rare use of glycopeptides in the local hospital (Klare et al 1993) suggested that hospitals may not be the only source of VRE. Besides their use in human chemotherapy, glycopeptides are also used as growth promoters in animal husbandry.

Avoparcin and its ergotropic use

Since 1975 the antibiotic avoparcin has been available as a feed additive in many countries (although not in the USA and Canada). As with other glycopeptides, avoparcin is not absorbed from the gut. Depending upon the livestock, 4–50 mg/kg of avoparcin is added to animal feed (Feed Additive Directive 70/524 of the EC). It was first licensed in 1975 and is now progressively used for feeding broiler chickens, turkeys, pigs, beef and dairy cattle, calves, sheep and goats.

As with bacitracin, tylosin and virginiamycin, the ergotropic (growth-stimulating) effect of avoparcin is thought to be due to a selective suppression of the Gram-positive bacterial gut flora, including enterococci. Although its precise mechanism of action is far from clear, it is thought to involve a reduction of the extent to which bile salts are decomposed by bacteria such as *E. faecium* (Feighner & Dashkevicz 1987).

Ergotropic use of avoparcin and selection for resistance

At the beginning of its ergotropic use, avoparcin at 1–2 mg/kg was shown to be effective in stimulating growth of poultry and reducing their enterococcal faecal flora (Dutta & Devriese 1982). Up to two years later no resistant enterococci had been detected (Dutta & Devriese 1984). These studies were hampered by a lack of analysis of enterococcal populations for resistant strains (no use of selective media containing avoparcin): a number of single isolates from plates without avoparcin were subjected to resistance determination.

When, in a later study, *Enterococcus* spp. were isolated from the gut flora of five non-medicated chickens, 8 of 20 isolates exhibited minimum inhibitory concentrations (MICs) for avoparcin of 10 mg/l; in one strain the MIC was ≥ 30 mg/l (Barrow

1989). Although there was no precise diagnostics of enterococcal species with respect to current taxonomy (see intrinsic resistance in E. *casseliflavus* and E. *gallinarum*) and no demonstration of the *vanA* gene, the possible emergence of VRE in broiler chickens cannot be excluded.

Studies performed in three European countries strongly suggest that avoparcin application selects for glycopeptide-resistant enterococci.

The first indications came from an in-depth analysis of dissemination of VRE in Great Britain. After the emergence of clinical VRE isolates in an Oxford hospital and the detection of VRE in faecal samples of both hospitalized and non-hospitalized patients (Jordens et al 1994), a broader investigation was performed by Bates et al (1993) on VRE from humans in the community and on VRE in farm animals and sewage samples. The E. *faecium* isolates were typed by ribotyping and 14 distinguishable patterns were found. Although ribotyping of E. *faecium* seems to be less discriminative than an *Sma*I macrorestriction pattern (Gordillo et al 1993), the different ribotypes suggest that a hospital origin of porcine VRE in this study is rather unlikely.

In our own study, we found glycopeptide-resistant E. *faecium* in samples of manure from a large pig farm and from a broiler chicken farm both using avoparcin, but not in manure from a farm with egg-laying chickens not receiving avoparcin. In addition to these data, VRE were isolated from slurry of another large avoparcin-using pig farm in Thuringia. In all VRE, cross-resistance to vancomycin, teicoplanin and avoparcin was found, independent of the ecological origin of the isolates.

All isolated VRE were of the *vanA* genotype as shown by PCR for the *vanA* gene and by demonstration of the 39 kDa cytoplasmic membrane protein as its product (Klare et al 1995a). VRE from different sources exhibited a variety of different *Sma*I macrorestriction patterns (Klare et al 1995a), which suggests a polyclonal nature of VRE. This was later confirmed by multilocus enzyme electrophoresis (Klare et al 1995b). There is obviously a wide spread of the *vanA* gene cluster among different E. *faecium* strains.

In our study, we used selective plates to look for VRE in animal faeces and slurry. We were unable to detect VRE in samples from 11 different farms in the vicinity of the provincial town Wernigerode and from six farms in the north of Baden-Württemberg, all of which did not use avoparcin or other antibiotics as growth promoters. A recent large-scale study in Denmark has confirmed our results (Aarestrup 1995): VRE were found in poultry faecal samples in six out of eight conventional farms that used avoparcin but not from poultry in six ecological farms which did not use antibiotics as feed additives at all.

Dissemination of VRE via the food chain

Contamination by the faecal flora of chicken broiler carcasses and meat during slaughtering and further processing cannot be completely avoided. It is therefore no surprise that we have found abundant VRE in the thawing liquid of commercially available poultry broilers and also in low quantities in five samples of raw minced meat from 13 different butcher's shops (see also Table 2). It is a custom to eat raw minced meat in this provincial area of Germany or to produce a smoked sausage from it which is then not heated any further before consumption.

However, no VRE were isolated from 29 meat samples originating from pigs reared without antibiotic feeding.

VRE in non-hospitalized humans

If VRE are disseminated via the food chain, they should occur more frequently among the community than originally thought. Bates et al (1994) found that three (2%) of 184 faecal samples from the community around Oxford were positive for VRE, and Gordts et al (1994) reported VRE in 22 (3.5%) of 636 faecal samples from patients entering a Belgian hospital. In another study in Charleroi, Belgium, seven of 40 people with no association to healthcare had VRE in their stools (J. van der Auwera, B. Murray & B. Leclercq, personal communication 1995). We have detected VRE (harbouring the *vanA* gene) in faeces from 12 of 100 non-hospitalized inhabitants of a provincial district in Germany (Table 2, for details see Klare et al 1995b).

If a gene conferring resistance to antibiotics has already become widely disseminated in the community, it is always difficult to refute the argument that this gene has been selected in hospital settings and has been brought to farm animals via contacts with humans and sewage. However, in the provincial German district in which our study was performed, an influence of hospitals is rather unlikely. Therapeutic use of glycopeptides is still exceptional in both of the district's hospitals, and VRE had not been isolated from clinical materials within the past five years (Table 2).

In conclusion, VRE seems to be widely distributed among different European countries. At present it is not known whether VRE are temporary passengers of the human gut, depending upon previous food uptake, or if they already have become a permanent constituent of the human gut flora. In contrast to the findings from Europe, no VRE were isolated from non-hospitalized humans in a study performed in Houston, Texas (B. Murray, personal communication). This may be related to the fact that no glycopeptides are licensed for animal feeding in the United States.

The data reviewed here strongly suggest that in addition to hospitals, animal husbandry also creates a large reservoir of VRE and thus a potential pool for the *vanA* gene.

Natural transfer of Tn*1546* coding for glycopeptide resistance appears to be rather frequent among *E. faecium* as suggested by the large number of distinct macrorestriction patterns found among VRE from identical ecological sources (Klare et al 1995a,b). Experimental conjugative transfer is also possible with *E. faecalis* (Uttley et al 1989) and was also demonstrated between *E. faecalis* and *Staphylococcus aureus* (Noble et al 1992). That a horizontal gene transfer between *S. aureus* and enterococci is possible under natural conditions is indicated by the high

TABLE 2 Occurrence of glycopeptide-resistant *E. faecium* (*vanA* mediated) outside hospitals in animals, in meat products and in faecal samples of non-hospitalized humans in a provincial district of Germany

Hospitals	Community	Food	Animal husbandry
District's two hospitals (A, B) each with ~700 beds and 12 000–15 000 in-patients per year[a]	100 non-hospitalized humans (inhabitants)	Samples of raw minced meat from 13 different producers	Large pig farm with ergotropic use of avoparcin
• no glycopeptide-resistant enterococci isolated from infections in humans from 1990 until now	• 12 faecal samples positive for glycopeptide resistant *E. faecium* (*vanA* mediated)	• 5 positive for glycopeptide-resistant *E. faecium* (*vanA* mediated)	• Glycopeptide-resistant *E. faecium* (*vanA* mediated) frequent in manure
~300 enterococcal strains assayed per year from hospitalized patients			11 small individual holdings of pigs in villages, no avoparcin use
			• No glycopeptide-resistant *E. faecium* in faecal samples

[a]Therapeutic use of glycopeptides in 1994: hospital A, 60 daily doses vancomycin (VM), 40 daily doses teicoplanin (TE), no oral applications; hospital B, 42 daily doses VM, 125 daily doses TE, no oral applications (for both hospitals this corresponds on average to 26 patients treated). (For details, see Klare et al 1995b.)

TABLE 3 Spread of plasmids carrying transposons-mediating streptothricin resistance among various bacterial populations in former Eastern Germany (Tschäpe 1994)

Origin	1982	1983	1984	1985	1986	1987
Gut flora of nourseothricin-fed pigs[a]	−	+	+	+	+	+
Gut flora of pig farm personnel[a]	−	−	+	+	+	+
Gut flora of family of pig farm personnel[a]	−	−	+	+	+	+
Gut flora of healthy adults[a]	−	−	−	+	+	+
Urinary tract infections[a] in humans	−	−	−	+	+	+
Shigella sonnei	−	−	−	−	−	+

[a]*E. coli.*

similarity of transposons encoding aminoglycoside resistance in *S. aureus* and in *E. faecalis* (Hodel-Christian & Murray 1991). A further expansion of pools of the *vanA* gene cluster also increases the risk of its spreading to staphylococci.

Further studies must show whether the ergotropic use of tylosin and of virginiamycin also select for the transfer of glycopeptide resistance in enterococci, since the *vanA* gene cluster and the *ermB* gene can be located on the same conjugative plasmid (Arthur & Courvalin 1993; G. Werner & W. Witte, unpublished data 1996).

Looking at the present situation with VRE, one is reminded of studies showing the spread of determinants conferring resistance to antibiotics which are only used in animal husbandry, and not in veterinary and animal chemotherapy.

Ergotropic use of a streptothricin antibiotic and spread of streptothricin resistance

In the former East Germany, the streptothricin antibiotic nourseothricin replaced oxytetracycline in animal feeding in 1983 and was used nation-wide for animal feeding only. No resistance was seen in Enterobacteriaceae from animals and humans at this time. The first occurrence of a transposon-coded resistance mechanism (streptothricin acetyltransferase) was observed two years later in *E. coli* from the gut flora of pigs. By the time its use was stopped after German reunification in 1990, resistance had spread to *E. coli* from the gut flora of pig farmers, further family members and also to *E. coli* from citizens of municipal communities and from urinary tract infections. The resistance determinants obviously spread in the absence of any selective pressure (Table 3).

Finally, the resistance determinant was detected in *Salmonella* and *Shigella* from cases of diarrhoea (Hummel et al 1986, Tschäpe 1994). Another example for a transfer of resistance determinants from animal husbandry to human pathogens is the

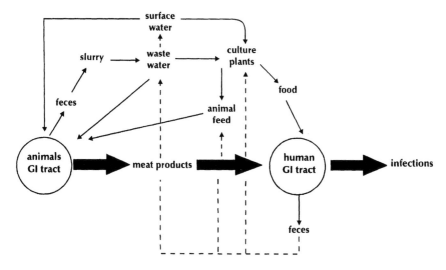

FIG. 1. Possible pathways of dissemination of antibiotic-resistant bacteria with the gastro-intestinal (GI) tract as the main reservoir between humans and animals.

determinant for aminoglycoside acetyltransferase IV, conferring cross-resistance to gentamicin and apramycin. In France, apramycin is exclusively used for chemotherapy in cattle. The resistance determinants were first observed in *E. coli* from animals, followed by strains from the environment; later they were found in *E. coli* able to cause infections in humans (Chaslus-Dancla et al 1989).

That a conjugative transfer of multidrug resistance plasmids between bacteria of different origin is also possible in natural microenvironments was recently demonstrated by Kruse & Sorum (1994). In conclusion, the use of antibiotics as feed additives creates potential for a reservoir of transferable resistance determinants. A permanent communication between this reservoir and reservoirs in the human body (above all the intestinal flora) is maintained with the food chain as the main route of transmission (Fig. 1). As the studies reviewed here illustrate, resistance determinants are able to spread horizontally and in the absence of detectable antibiotic selective pressure. Although it is difficult to quantify the extent of this spread, antibiotic use in animal feeding obviously contributes to the development of resistance in human bacterial pathogens.

References

Aarestrup FM 1995 Occurrence of glycopeptide resistance among *Enterococcus faecium* isolates from conventional and ecological poultry farms. Microb Drug Res 1:255–257

Arthur M, Courvalin P 1993 Genetics and mechanisms of glycopeptide resistance in enterococci. Antimicrob Agents Chemother 37:1563–1571

Bates J, Jordens Z, Selkon JB 1993 Evidence for animal origin of vancomycin resistant enterococci. Lancet 342:490–491

Bates J, Jordens Z, Griffith DT 1994 Farm animals as a putative reservoir for vancomycin resistant enterococcal infection in man. J Antimicrob Chemother 34:507–514

Barrow PA 1989 Further observations on the effect of feeding diets containing avoparcin on the excretion of Salmonellas by experimentally infected chickens. Epidemiol Infect 102:239–252

Bingen EH, Denamur E, Lambert-Zechovsky NJ, Elion J 1991 Evidence for the genetic unrelatedness of nosocomial vancomycin-resistant *Enterococcus faecium* strains in a pediatric hospital. J Clin Microbiol 29:1888–1892

Centers for Disease Control 1993 Nosocomial enterococci resistant to vancomycin — United States 1989–1993. Morb Mortal Wkly Rep 42:597–599

Centers for Disease Control 1995 Recommendations for preventing the spread of vancomycin resistance. Morb Mortal Wkly Rep 44:RR12

Chaslus-Dancla E, Glupczynski J, Gerbaud G, Lagorce M, Lafont JP, Courvalin P 1989 Detection of apramycin resistant Enterobacteriaceae in hospital isolates. FEMS Microbiol Lett 61:261–266

Courvalin P 1990 Resistance of enterococci to glycopeptides. Antimicrob Agents Chemother 34:2291–2296

Dutta GN, Devriese LA 1982 Susceptibility of faecal streptococci of poultry origin to nine growth promoting agents. Appl Environ Microbiol 44:832–837

Dutta GN, Devriese LA 1984 Observations on the *in vitro* sensitivity and resistance of gram positive intestinal bacteria of farm animals to growth promoting antimicrobial agents. J Appl Bacteriol 56:117–123

Evers S, Sahun BF, Courvalin P 1993 The vanB gene of vancomycin resistant *Enterococcus faecalis* V583 is structurally related to genes encoding D-Ala-D-Ala ligases and glycopeptide resistance proteins VanA and VanC. Gene 124:143–144

Feighner SD, Dashkevicz MD 1987 Subtherapeutic levels of antibiotics in poultry feeds and their effects on weight gain, feed efficiency, and bacterial cholyltaurine hydrolase activity. Appl Environ Microbiol 53:331–336

Frieden TR, Munsiff S, Low DE et al 1993 Emergence of vancomycin-resistant enterococci in New York City. Lancet 342:76–79

Gordillo ME, Singh KV, Murray BE 1993 Comparison of ribotyping and pulsed-field gel electrophoresis for subspecies differentiation of strains of *Enterococcus faecalis*. J Clin Microbiol 31:1571–1574

Gordts B, Clayes K, Jannes H, van Landuyt HW 1994 Are vancomycin resistant enterococci (VRE) normal inhabitants of the GI tract of hospitalized patients? 34th Interscience Conference on Antimicrobial Agents and Chemotherapy, Abstract J151

Helmuth R, Bulling E (eds) 1985 Criteria and methods for the microbiological evaluation of growth promoters in animal feeds. Bundesgesundheitsamt, Berlin

Hodel-Christian SL, Murray BE 1991 Characterization of the gentamicin resistance transposon Tn*5281* from *Enterococcus faecalis* and comparison to staphylococcal transposons Tn*4001* and Tn*4301*. Antimicrob Agents Chemother 35:1147–1152

Hummel R, Tschäpe H, Witte W 1986 Spread of plasmid mediated nourseothricin resistance due to antibiotic use in animal husbandry. J Basic Microbiol 26:461–466

Jordens JZ, Bates J, Griffiths DT 1994 Faecal carriage and nosocomial spread of vancomycin-resistant *E. faecium*. J Antimicrob Chemother 34:515–528

Klare I, Heier H, Claus H, Witte W 1993 Environmental strains of *Enterococcus faecium* with inducible high level resistance to glycopeptides. FEMS Microbiol Lett 106:23–90

Klare I, Heier H, Claus H, Reissbrodt R, Witte W 1995a *vanA*-mediated high-level glycopeptide resistance in *Enterococcus faecium* from animal husbandry. FEMS Microbiol Lett 125:165–172

Klare I, Heier H, Claus H et al 1995b *Enterococcus faecium* strains with *vanA*-mediated high-level glycopeptide resistance isolated from animal foodstuffs and fecal samples of humans in the community. Microb Drug Res 1:265–272

Kruse H, Sorum H 1994 Transfer of multiple drug resistance plasmids between bacteria of diverse origin in natural microenvironments. Appl Environ Microbiol 60:4015–4021

Levy SB, Fitzgerald GB, Macone AB 1976a Spread of antibiotic resistance plasmids from chicken to chicken and from chicken to man. Nature 260:40

Levy SB, Fitzgerald GB, Macone AB 1976b Changes in intestinal flora of farm personnel after introduction of tetracycline-supplemented feed on a farm. New Engl J Med 295:583–588

Navarro F, Courvalin P 1994 Analysis of genes encoding D-alanine-D-alanine ligase related enzymes in *Enterococcus casseliflavus* and *Enterococcus flavescens*. Antimicrob Agents Chemother 38:1788–1793

Noble WC, Virani Z, Cree RGA 1992 Co-transfer of vancomycin and other resistance genes from *Enterococcus faecalis* NCTC 12201 to *Staphylococcus aureus*. FEMS Microbiol Lett 93:195–198

Torres C, Reguera JA, Sanmartin MJ, Perez-Diaz JC, Baquero F 1994 *vanA*-mediated vancomycin-resistant *Enterococcus* spp. in sewage. J Antimicrob Chemother 33:553–561

Tschäpe H 1994 The spread of plasmids as a function of bacterial adaptability. FEMS Microbiol Lett 15:23–32

Uttley AHC, George RC, Naidoo J et al 1989 High level vancomycin resistant enterococci causing hospital infections. Epidemiol Infect 103:173–181

WHO 1995 WHO Scientific Working Group on Monitoring and Management of Bacterial Resistance to Antimicrobial Agents (CDSI B VI). World Health Organization, Geneva

DISCUSSION

Huovinen: How do you explain the fact that in the USA avoparcin has never been used and yet there are these vancomycin-resistant strains?

Witte: I can't, but I can speculate. In the USA cephalosporins are much more widely used. Post-antibiotic enterocolitis is more frequent in the USA than in central European hospitals, and it was always thought that the drug of choice in post-antibiotic enterocolitis was vancomycin. The CDC recommended last year that this use be reduced and that vancomycin should only be used in life-threatening conditions. This might explain the higher frequency in the USA.

Levy: The data look clear that in the animal population the use of avoparcin has created vancomycin resistance among enterococci. The papers from Oxford by Janice Bates and colleagues tell us that there are the same kinds of enterococci in humans and animals (Bates et al 1994). The topic of our meeting is the origin of resistance determinants. Can we say that the problem of vancomycin resistance in the USA has anything to do with the reservoir of avoparcin-resistant enterococci in Europe? We have not been able to find that reservoir in the USA. It is clear that 10 years of use of avoparcin — that was considered an animal-only antibiotic — has created a reservoir of resistant enterococci of potential threat to humans.

Davies: Why is it necessary to use avoparcin in the USA? Isn't there enough selective pressure for glycopeptide resistance from use in the hospital! I should remind you that vancomycin, like many antibiotics, is not pure; it contains DNA from the producing organism and it is possible that this contributes to the development of antibiotic resistance (Webb & Davies 1993).

Levy: In the USA we use a lot of vancomycin, whereas Europe uses far less. There is this therefore this important difference — a reservoir of resistant organisms in the animal population in Europe but not in humans, whereas this is a big nosocomial problem in the USA where 20–30% of a hospital's antibiotic budget may be devoted to vancomycin.

Piddock: We've shown that ciprofloxacin-resistant campylobacter were introduced to the UK from other parts of the European Community (Gaunt & Piddock 1996). I see no reason why food couldn't have gone from Europe to the USA and thus transferred VRE in this way.

Witte: We have thought of that possibility, but we were informed that besides frozen pigs from Denmark, no other meat is imported to the USA from Europe. However, fast food chains import beef from Latin American countries, where avoparcin is used for fattening cows.

Levy: The few studies that have been done in the USA have not found avoparcin-resistant enterococci associated with meat. However, there was a recent letter in *ASM News* last month where a student found a vancomycin-resistant enterococcus in dog food!

Cohen: One thing that's always troubled me about VRE outbreaks in the USA is that in many hospitals resistance is not clonal. When you subtype, the VREs from an outbreak are often a combination of different strains. These outbreaks may represent mixed modes of transmission — acquisition outside the hospital of various strains selected by cephalosporin and vancomycin use in the hospital coupled with person-to-person transmission from inappropriate infection control practices.

Summers: I want to ask about the streptothricin resistance study. You said something about the association with Tn7, which is a transposon. You used the term 'in the absence of selective pressure', presumably meaning in the absence of streptothricin administration. Were there other antibiotics administered, and was there any assessment made of the genetic linkage of the streptothricin resistance alleles to other antibiotics used?

Witte: When we looked for transposons of the Tn7 family at the position where normally the dihydrofolate reductase gene is located, we found streptothricin acetyltransferase in streptothricin resistance transposons. On that transposon there is also a determinant for spectinomycin resistance. Spectinomycin was never available in former Eastern Germany. We have not looked for linkage with other resistance determinants.

Summers: I think genetic linkage absolutely must be considered and evaluated as a possible explanation for gratuitous selection of linked resistances.

Hall: The emergence of that streptothricin resistance gene, *sat1/2*, is interesting, because that gene, though not expressed, is found in Tn7. Tn7 was first isolated prior to 1983, so the gene existed when no one was using the antibiotic streptothricin. Tn7 became widespread; presumably because it contains a trimethoprim resistance gene and it is selected by trimethoprim use.

Levy: Of critical note to the study was that no streptothricin was being used in the people. Thus, resistance would not have been selected by human use. Yet urinary tract isolates of *E. coli* from the same community where the animals were fed had this resistance. It was of no distinct consequence to therapy. It appears that this particular Tn7 moved from the pigs to the farm personnel, to the families of the people working on the farms, to the people in the community. This is the only prospective study that I know which shows how rapidly an unselected marker can move from animals to people.

Summers: The point I was making was that this marker is unselected by the specific antibiotic under study, but it could have been selected for by another antibiotic. We have this paradox: we have agreed that the resistant environmental bacteria get in there and colonize people and they hang out there. In other contexts we're saying the exogenous flora passing through is transient, unable to compete with the person's indigenous flora and colonize. We need to resolve whether and when one or the other outcome is true. I think one of the underlying factors in this might simply be genetic linkage. An incoming bug will have a better chance of colonizing if it's carrying genes for resistance to a drug which the person is taking. But this resistance may be linked to lots of others and all of them will stay.

Baquero: I am an advisor to a scientific committee for animal nutrition in Brussels. There has been a lot of discussion about this issue because of the economic consequences of the elimination of avoparcin from animal feeding. The sorts of figures they are talking about are that if avoparcin is no longer used the cost of food will increase by 25%. This brings us round to the discussion of risk assessment: how important is the problem? The risk that I proposed to the committee is (at least) one death per million inhabitants per year in Europe due to VRE. One problem is that so many people are now low level carriers of VRE that whether or not avoparcin is used in animals will probably now make little difference.

Threlfall: Over the years this has been a major question. Even now certain pharmaceutical companies and animal health organizations still use the argument that the use of antibiotics in animals has had little or no impact on resistance in humans. In closed committee meetings they are claiming, for example, that multiresistant salmonella strains have been spread to animals through human sewage spread on the farms. This is a vexed question which needs serious discussion.

Davies: Wolfgang Witte mentioned that virginiamycins are used in animal feed. This is interesting because the virginiamycins are cross-resistant to all of the streptogramins, including new derivatives that have just been introduced, one of which is supposed to be a leading candidate for treating vancomycin-resistant MRSA should it arise. Resistance to virginiamycin in animals is already abundant, so this unhappy situation has been well established in advance of human use of the antibiotic!

Levy: There are unpublished data from the USA showing that the isolates from virginiamycin-treated animals are resistant to the new streptogramins, so the cross-resistance is there. In view of these findings one could ask why we are wasting these antibiotics on growth promotion when there are other options. Fernando Baquero stated that members of the animal nutrition committee of the EU are worried about a 25% increase in food prices if antibiotics are no longer fed to animals. I find this figure excessive. Denmark didn't seem to worry when they banned this use.

Witte: I don't know where that figure of 25% comes from.

Baquero: These data come from the companies marketing avoparcin and tylosin.

Hall: The real question is, are there satisfactory data proving that antibiotics have any growth promotion effect?

Levy: There is always a mix between what portion of the antibiotic usage is for growth promotion and what is for prophylaxis. If you look at the data there is a clear growth promotion effect — less now then there was earlier because of better rearing — but it's in the range of a few percent. That is why many companies in the USA are voluntarily moving away from this use.

Piddock: To use an antibiotic in animal husbandry you have to get a licence, and you can get a licence for certain uses just the same as you can for human use. Many of the licences being granted now are for veterinary use only — in other words to treat ill animals, not for prophylaxis or food additives. The trouble is, how does one treat one or two chickens in a chicken house of several thousand? It's easy to see how these things get justified on a veterinary ticket when the use is not really veterinary at all. In the UK before enrofloxacin was licensed, several farmers were taken to court for importing enrofloxacin prior to getting a licence. However, I cannot see anybody being prosecuted for using it in an inappropriate manner because it's going to be so difficult to prove.

I think it's very unlikely that once a product is licensed, the licence will be withdrawn. In most European countries, politics combined with financial pressures upon farmers and the pharmaceutical industry are such that this will not happen. As Fernando said, it is not cost effective, when you don't have very many people actually dying of the antibiotic-resistant organism. The other point frequently raised is that it is almost impossible to prove that the antibiotic-resistant bacteria not only have come from the animal but have caused the infection from which a patient has died. That is what many companies hang their hat on.

Cohen: A societal decision about what costs are tolerated is critical. When we discussed this issue in the 1970s, a main point was whether or not use of certain drugs would increase the price of poultry by a few cents a pound. The public was never given a choice to make a decision as to whether they would be willing to pay 'X' amount for withdrawing certain drugs from use. In fact, what tends to happen is that often these decisions are made on the basis of public outrage: some adverse event occurs, often an outbreak of disease that is linked to a practice, that pushes the decision out of a cost–benefit discussion into a political one. Very often that's when there's movement in these kinds of issues.

References

Bates J, Jordens Z, Griffith DT 1994 Farm animals as a putative reservoir for vancomycin resistant enterococcal infection in man. J Antimicrob Chemother 34:507–514

Gaunt PN, Piddock LJV 1996 Ciprofloxacin resistant campylobacter in humans: an epidemiological and laboratory study. J Antimicrob Chemother 37:747–757

Webb V, Davies J 1993 Antibiotic preparations contain DNA—a source of drug resistance genes. Antimicrob Agents Chemother 37:2379–2384

The effect of monitoring of antibiotic use on decreasing antibiotic resistance in the hospital

Helen Giamarellou and Anastasia Antoniadou

Infectious Diseases Section, Athens University School of Medicine, 1st Department of Propedeutic Medicine, Laiko, General Hospital, GR 115 27, Athens, Greece

Abstract. In Greece, antibiotic over-consumption and high resistance rates run in parallel. In the spring of 1989 surveillance of 12 500 Gram-negative strains, derived from 55 hospitals from all over Greece, revealed that resistance rates of *Pseudomonas aeruginosa*, *Enterobacter* spp., *Klebsiella* spp. and *Acinetobacter* spp. to antimicrobial agents introduced after 1985 exceeded 50%. As a consequence, the application of (1) rules of hospital hygiene, (2) educational small group programs, and (3) an antibiotic policy aiming to restrict antibiotic use, was decided in Laiko General Hospital. Since 1989, imipenem, the newer quinolones, vancomycin, aztreonam and third-generation cephalosporins were only ordered to the hospital pharmacy after completion of a specific request form, which since 1991 has been more detailed and which can be signed only by physicians with interest in infectious diseases. In 1991, in cooperation with the pharmacy, an audit program was added requiring a final inspection of the already approved request forms by an infectious diseases specialist. Any disagreement was discussed with the physicians in charge. Consumption data were analysed monthly and discussed with each department. Newer antibiotic consumption in a selected month (November) of three consecutive years, before (1991) and after the application of the audit program (1992–1995) has been analysed. Results reveal a decrease in consumption of restricted antibiotics, especially in surgical departments and in kidney transplantation units, without simultaneous increase in consumption of the non-restricted compounds. Since 1994, resistance has decreased remarkably. However, the resistance of quinolones is increasing steeply. Consequently, for the last 12 months quinolones have been removed from the hospital formulary. An audit program requires close co-operation of physicians, pharmacists and, particularly, of surgeons, in the application of a correct prophylaxis regimen. It seems to be efficacious in reducing both resistance rates and total antibiotic consumption.

1997 Antibiotic resistance: origins, evolution, selection and spread. Wiley, Chichester (Ciba Foundation Symposium 207) p 76–92

The emergence of resistance to antimicrobial agents is now a major problem in both the hospital and the community (Levy 1990, Murray 1991, Cohen 1992, Neu 1992, Kunin 1993, Kresken et al 1994). Bacteria employ a variety of strategies to avoid the inhibitory effects of antibiotics, and have evolved highly efficient means for the dissemination of resistance traits. The result has been the emergence of multidrug-resistant pathogens such as penicillin-resistant pneumococci, vancomycin-resistant enterococci, methicillin-resistant staphylococci, as well as a variety of multiresistant Gram-negative organisms (Murray 1991). Among the latter, *Pseudomonas aeruginosa*, *Acinetobacter baumannii* and *Enterobacter cloacae* usually predominate with high morbidity and mortality in hospital-acquired infections, particularly those acquired in intensive care units (Giamarellou et al 1986, Holmberg et al 1987). Control of antibiotic-resistant pathogens will provide a major challenge for both the medical community and society in general. The implication of a failure to meet this challenge would be 'a worldwide calamity' (Kunin 1993) while it has been predicted that 'if the currently effective antibiotics are not preserved or newer effective antimicrobials are not developed, and the transmission of drug-resistant organism curtailed, the post-antimicrobial era may be rapidly approaching, in which infectious diseases wards housing untreatable conditions will again be seen' (Cohen 1992). Infectious disease 'prophets' are now predicting the forthcoming 'end of antibiotics' (Begley 1994).

For the time being, there is no doubt that despite the existence of >150 antimicrobial agents, a person can die as a result of a multiresistant bacterial infection (Neu 1992). Despite the rumours that multiresistant microorganisms may lose their pathogenic potential, Holmberg et al (1987), after reviewing 87 reports on nosocomial and community acquired infections, have stated that 'the mortality, the likelihood of hospitalization and the length of hospital stay, were at least twice as great for patients infected with resistant strains as for those infected with drug-susceptible strains of the same bacteria'.

Among the unwanted consequences of antimicrobial therapy are adverse reactions, emergence of drug-resistant microorganisms, predisposition to secondary infections and the increased cost of medical care. On the other hand, there is a consensus that antibiotics are used excessively, that documentation of why they are used is often lacking in medical records, and that control measures could lead to significant financial savings.

It has been shown that roughly one-half of antibiotic use is 'inappropriate', whether in hospitals, outpatient clinics, or extended-care facilities. At least for the hospital setting, seven lines of evidence have linked antimicrobial misuse and overuse with antimicrobial resistance in hospital bacteria (McGowan 1983): (1) antimicrobial resistance is more prevalent in bacterial strains causing nosocomial infection than in organisms from community-acquired cases; (2) during outbreaks, patients with resistant strains are more likely to have received prior antibiotic therapy than control patients; (3) changes in antimicrobial usage lead to parallel changes in prevalence of resistance; (4) areas within the hospital having the highest usage of antimicrobials also have the highest prevalence of antibiotic-resistant bacteria (special care units); (5) an increasing likelihood of colonization or infection with resistant organisms occurs with increasing duration of exposure to antimicrobials in the hospital; (6) inadequate dosage of antimicrobials leads to greater likelihood of superinfection or colonization with resistant organisms; and (7) antimicrobial usage in hospitals is extensive and antibiotics are present in the hospital environment. As a result, both patients and hospital employees are exposed to antimicrobials.

The magnitude of the problem was evident when the Infectious Diseases Society of America (IDSA) in the effort to improve antibiotic use almost ten years ago sent a questionnaire to its members (Kunin 1985). Of 881 who responded, only 4.6% were in favour of the 'don't interfere' attitude, while 85.4% agreed on education efforts, 87.3% on controlled antibiotic use and 64.3% to restrain promotion!

Strategies to improve antibiotic use

On the basis of the evidence outlined above, several policies and strategies have been considered in the effort to improve antibiotic usage (Gould 1988, Marr 1988, Bryan 1989, Quintilliani et al 1991). The following have been considered as effective.

Education

Although education should be considered as the cornerstone of any program, several studies have suggested that efforts to influence the antibiotic prescribing habits of house officers by education were ineffective in both inpatient and outpatient settings. The most useful educational sessions appear to be 'one-on-one instruction' or 'group consultation' with an infectious diseases expert. However, education might focus not so much on which antibiotics should be used but rather on how to make an accurate diagnosis of infection.

The hospital formulary

Control of the hospital formulary continues to be a powerful method for curbing the tendency for the newer agents to displace older, still-effective ones.

Ordering policies

Examples of effective ordering policies include: (1) standards for prophylactic antibiotics for surgery, which has long been identified as the most frequent area of 'inappropriate' use of antibiotics; (2) automatic stop orders; (3) the requirement for written justification through special order forms; (4) rotating policies; and (5) the use of expensive, specialized agents to be a privilege of infectious diseases consultants.

Drug utilization review

An approach applicable to all hospitals is to ask that each clinical service designate one infectious diseases consultant to review the use of antibiotics. Their tasks include: (1) analysis of pharmacy expenditures for antibiotics; (2) audit of use of individual drugs;

(3) detailed analysis of individual cases; (4) survey of usage in individual services; (5) survey of all orders for surgical prophylaxis; (6) survey of therapeutic use according to diagnosis; (7) approval of clinical trials; and (8) ongoing surveillance of all antibiotic use.

Restriction policies

These require that certain drugs be approved by designated physicians — mainly infectious diseases specialists. Usually, three categories of drugs are considered: (1) 'restricted' i.e. removed from the formulary for routine use; (2) 'controlled' i.e. subjected to automatic stop orders; and (3) 'non-restricted'. Many studies have indicated that restriction policies are very effective.

Control of laboratory susceptibility testing data

Selective reporting of laboratory susceptibility test results has been considered as a powerful means of influencing prescribing habits.

Limitation of contact time between pharmaceutical representatives and physicians

It has been enforced only sporadically mainly because they are considered as helpful 'colleagues' who provide quick information, guest speakers, funds for education and research, and travel grants.

Implementation of rules of hygiene

The implementation of rules of hygiene, particularly hand-washing, to restrict the spread of multiresistant strains in the hospital environment is of extreme importance.

The antimicrobial agents team

In several US hospitals, the 'antimicrobial agents team' consisting of an infectious diseases physician, an infection control practitioner, a clinical microbiologist and a clinical pharmacist, has been found extremely important for the organization and implementation of rational antibiotic policies.

The Greek strategy for improving antibiotic use

In Greece in the 1980s extremely high resistance rates were reported, which ran in parallel with extremely high antibiotic consumption (Tables 1–3) (Giamarellou et al 1986). Particularly in Laiko General Hospital, the main University teaching hospital with a 500 bed capacity, antibiotic consumption in the hospitalized patients ranged in the 1985–89 period from 62–78% with the highest rates in General Surgery and Urology departments (75–100%). The main overuse involved >7 d antibiotic

TABLE 1 **Percentage of resistance in 2164 Gram-negatives derived from blood culture isolates (ESGAR 1987)**

	Sweden	Great Britain	Spain	Germany	Belgium	France	Italy	Portugal	Greece
Cefotaxime	2	1	2	0	5	7	20	7	32
Ceftazidime	2	3	2	5	5	4	5	11	20
Netilmicin	2	3	11	9	21	16	22	32	35
Amikacin	3	4	5	8	11	8	13	3	41
Imipenem	2	2	0.4	2	0.8	1	2	4	0.5
Ciprofloxacin	0.6	1	1	1	0.8	8	0.7	6	3
Aztreonam	3	2	2	9	9	10	10	8	29

prophylaxis, while one-third to half of antibiotic prescription involved third-generation cephalosporins, imipenem, newer quinolones and vancomycin.

Antibiotic overuse and abuse in Greece, both in the community and the hospital setting, has been attributed to the following reasons:

(1) Doctors tend to prescribe more antibiotics than necessary: they give antimicrobials where they are not indicated, use drugs of a broader spectrum than is necessary and continue therapy longer than required.
(2) Prophylaxis, especially in surgery, is unjustified in the vast majority of the patients and when indicated is very rarely given perioperatively.

TABLE 2 **Resistance rates to several antimicrobial agents of 5454 Gram-negative isolates from 55 Greek hospitals during a three month period (Spring 1989)**

Antimicrobial agent	Pseudomonas aeruginosa No. 2183	Acinetobacter spp. No. 662	Enterobacter spp. No. 809	Klebsiella pneumoniae No. 1800
Cephalothin	—	—	95%	63%
Cefotaxime	—	—	77%	51%
Ceftazidime	31%	92%	67%	46%
Imipenem	14%	1.1%	4.2%	0.5%
Ciprofloxacin	26%	59.6%	13%	10%
Amikacin	44%	91%	51%	45%
Gentamicin	45%	83%	43%	36%
Tobramycin	42%	84%	71%	55%
Netilmicin	61%	90%	66%	45%

TABLE 3 Cephalosporin (Ceph) and newer quinolone (Q) consumption in Greece compared with other European countries

Year	Greece		Denmark		Ireland		Norway		Sweden[a]
	Ceph	Q	Ceph	Q	Ceph	Q	Ceph	Q	Ceph
1990	2.8	0.8	0.1	0.1	0.4	0.7	0.3	0.0	0.6
1991	2.6	1.0	0.1	0.2	0.3	0.6	0.3	0.1	0.6
1992	2.9	1.2	0.1	0.3	0.3	0.3	0.3	0.1	0.7

Numbers represent defined daily dose/1000 inhabitants per day.
[a]No data on quinolone consumption in Sweden were available.

(3) Microbiologists have a share in the blame: they often report the isolation of obvious commensals and worse, give sensitivities. For multi-sensitive pathogens they report sensitivities to newer, potent antibiotics.

(4) The patients themselves or their relatives insist on an antibiotic prescription and much too often the doctor yields to the pressure. The patients often listen to a friend's suggestion or they follow their own initiative and buy antibiotics over the counter for self-administration.

(5) The pharmacists are happy to comply. The Greek law prohibits antibiotic sale over the counter but there is no control whatsoever to detect and punish this practice.

(6) The pharmaceutical industry is highly active and very successful in their marketing of antibiotics in Greece.

Since 1990, an antibiotic restriction policy program was implemented by the Infection Control Committee at Laiko General Hospital in Athens, applied mainly by the Antibiotic Team (composed of an infectious diseases physician, a clinical microbiologist and a pharmacist), on the following bases:

(1) The need for optimal antimicrobial therapy for the benefit of the patient.

(2) The need to decrease the preponderance of multiresistant pathogens and to protect newer antibiotics from the development of resistance.

(3) The fact that in the near future the development of promising new antibacterial agents active against multiresistant pathogens seems very unlikely.

(4) The need to reduce the cost without diminishing medical services quality.

(5) Resistance elements can be lost when selective antibiotic pressure is removed and susceptible organisms do eventually return to colonize the ecological site (Cohen 1992, Neu 1992).

The program was also supplemented by the application of rules of hospital hygiene (particularly of hand washing and appropriate use of gloves), educational programs for

Name of patient.....................

Hospital Clinic....................... Admission Date...........

Type of Infection..

Underlying diseases(s)..

....

Isolated pathogen(s)...

Susceptibilities...

....

Preceded administration of antibiotics

    No ☐   Yes ☐

    Type of administered antibiotic(s)..

Justification of request ....

....

Anticipated duration of therapy : Days(≤ 5).......................................

Date...................

Physician   in charge Signature   Infectious Disease Inspector Signature

FIG. 1.   Example of the restricted antibiotic order form from Laiko General Hospital pharmacy.

small groups of physicians belonging to different clinics, 'consensus agreements' regarding mainly perioperative surgical prophylaxis, febrile neutropenia, and nosocomial pneumonia, and limited susceptibility reporting from the Central Diagnostic Microbiology Lab. According to the applied restricted antibiotic policies program, since January of 1989, all third- and fourth-generation cephalosporins, aztreonam, imipenem, the newer quinolones and vancomycin were ordered to the pharmacy only after physicians had completed a restricted antibiotic order form (Fig. 1), which had also been inspected and signed by the hospital infectious diseases clinicians or by physicians with a proven interest in infectious diseases (one for each hospital clinic). The immediate results of the program are shown in Table 4. It is remarkable that restricted antibiotic consumption was reduced by 80% without any lethal event attributed to restricted policies. Between 1989 and 1991, restricted

TABLE 4 The effect of a restricted antibiotic policies program on antibiotic consumption

| Restricted antibiotic | Number of patients on restricted antibiotics | | | | |
	January 1988 (Control[a])	September 1989	January 1990	March 1990	June 1990
Vancomycin	118	32	15	16	15
Imipenem	102	28	22	32	13
Ceftazidime	150	60	43	54	26
Total	370	120	80	102	54

[a]Consumption without restriction.

antibiotic use ranged between 4.2–7.0% among the hospitalized patients versus 29% in the control month of January 1988.

Because the Antibiotic Team had the impression that antibiotic usage could be improved further, in November 1992 an audit program in close cooperation with the pharmacy was applied. Three times a week, an infectious diseases physician (who rotated monthly) audited the antibiotic restriction order forms, before the pharmacy had delivered the required antibiotics. Whenever an order form was incomplete, or the provided justification for requiring any restricted antibiotic seemed irrational, the infectious diseases physician visited the clinics and discussed the case with the resident doctors. Also, every two months the Antibiotic Team organized separate scientific meetings for each clinic during which, in front of the staff and the residents, all irrational order forms were discussed. Such meetings provoked large-scale discussion and were considered to be the most effective educational program on antibiotic use.

After the introduction of the audit program a further significant reduction in restricted antibiotics was observed (Table 5). In the mean time, imipenem and vancomycin were considered as indispensable antibiotics only for treating multiresistant *Acinetobacter baumannii*, methicillin-resistant *Staphylococcus aureus*, sepsis syndrome and septic shock.

It has been estimated that antibiotics should be given to less than 30% of hospitalized patients (McGowan 1983). It is of interest that despite the fear that restriction of advanced antibiotics might increase the consumption of non-restricted antibiotics, in Laiko General Hospital all antibiotics use was reduced by more than 50%, total consumption ranging between 32% and 38.5%. As shown in Table 5, the reported reduction was mainly attributed to implementation of correct prophylaxis guidelines in the surgery departments, where one perioperative dose of either a first- or second-generation cephalosporin was administered in clean-contaminated operations.

TABLE 5 Consumption of restricted antimicrobials in the different clinics of Laiko General Hospital

Clinic	Number of patients on restricted antibiotics			
	November 1991 (no audit)	November 1991 (with audit)	November 1993 (with audit)	February 1995 (with audit)
General surgery	12.2%	3%	0.9%	0.7%
Urology	2.7%	0.3%	0.9%	1%
Orthopaedics	8.4%	1.9%	3.3%	2.5%
Transplant unit	19%	18%	7%	7.7%
Nephrology	19.2%	15%	17%	10%

After three years of applying the audit program, there has been a significant reduction in the resistance rates of several classes of antibiotic. In particular, for *P. aeruginosa*, a major nosocomial threat, resistance to ceftazidime was reduced from 45% to 8%, while for imipenem it remained as low as it was before the latter antibiotic was introduced into the Greek market ($\sim 3\%$). Interestingly, although aminoglycosides as a group were not restricted, their prescription in the hospital, due to the introduction of the newer β-lactams and the fear of nephrotoxicity, was minimal, confined only to septic or profoundly neutropenic patients. Mean resistance rates, which before 1990 were 55% and 85% for amikacin and gentamicin, respectively, were decreased to 12% and 19%. However, it should be pointed out that resistance to quinolones was not influenced by the antibiotic policy program. This was constantly increasing, with levels of 35%, 20% and 31% for *P. aeruginosa*, *Escherichia coli* and *Klebsiella pneumoniae*, observed respectively, in spring 1995. Consequently, the Antibiotic Team decided that quinolones should be totally restricted in the hospital, and should be prescribed only in cases where a pathogen is exclusively susceptible to this class of antimicrobials. The results of this restriction are pending.

Finally, it should be pointed out that before the application of any antibiotic policy program, knowledge of the underlying resistance mechanisms and particularly of the existence of plasmid-mediated determinants is extremely important (Giamarellou et al 1986). After having applied an antibiotic-restriction policy in a tertiary University Hospital in Athens, our experience has taught us the following:

(1) Given the enthusiasm of those who are going to apply it, we have shown that an audit program can be extremely successful in decreasing antibiotic resistance rates and cost containment.

(2) Since doctors are often pressured by pharmaceutical representatives to consider the newest and most expensive antibiotics, the implementation of such a program requires continuous audit and follow-up.

(3) The involvement of an infectious diseases physician, who should be highly respected in the hospital, is indispensable since clinicians and, in particular, surgeons are not eager to obey the recommendations of microbiologists regarding antibiotic prescribing.

(4) Cooperation with the pharmacy and the microbiology laboratory is essential.

(5) Education of doctors is successful only in the small group format and it should be on-going.

After all, physicians should remember that diagnosis of infection has the priority, and that their antibiotic prescription habit is an indicator of their self-esteem. The time has come for the medical profession to restrict its insistence on clinical freedom to prescribe what it likes and when it likes (Gould 1988). No other group of drugs, when misused, has such an effect on society, not only through the costs incurred, but also by the effects on bacterial resistance that may lead physicians and their patients into the 'post-antibiotic era'.

References

Begley S 1994 The end of antibiotics. Newsweek, March 28, p 39–42

Bryan CS 1989 Strategies to improve antibiotic use. Infect Dis Clin N Am 3:723–734

Cohen ML 1992 Epidemiology of drug resistance: implications for a post-antimicrobial era. Science 257:1050–1055

ESGAR (European Study Group on Antibiotic Resistance) 1987 In vitro susceptibility to aminoglycoside antibiotics in blood and urine isolates consecutively collected in twenty-nine European laboratories. Eur J Clin Microbiol 6:378–385

Giamarellou H, Touliatou K, Koratzanis G et al 1986 Nosocomial consequences of antibiotic usage. Scan J Infect Dis (suppl) 49:182–188

Gould JM 1988 Control of antibiotic use in the United Kingdom. J Antimicrob Chemother 22:395–401

Holmberg SD, Solomon SL, Blake PA 1987 Health and economic impacts on antimicrobial resistance. Rev Infect Dis 9:1065–1078

Kresken M, Hafner D, Mittermayer H, Verbist L, Bergogne-Berezin E, Giamarellou H 1994 Prevalence of fluoroquinolone resistance in Europe. Infection (suppl 2) 22:90–98

Kunin CM 1985 The responsibility of the infectious disease community for the optimal use of antimicrobial agents. J Infect Dis 181:388–398

Kunin CM 1993 Resistance to antimicrobial drugs: a worldwide calamity. Ann Intern Med 118:557–559

Levy SB 1990 Starting life resistance free. N Engl J Med 323:335–337

Marr JJ, Moffett HL, Kunin CM 1988 Guidelines for improving the use of antimicrobial agents in hospitals: a statement by the Infectious Diseases Society of America. J Infect Dis 157:869–876

McGowan JE 1983 Antimicrobial resistance in hospital organisms and its relation to antibiotic use. Rev Infect Dis 5:1033–1048

Murray BE 1991 New aspects of antimicrobial resistance and the resulting therapeutic dilemmas. J Infect Dis 163:1185–1194

Neu HC 1992 The crisis of antibiotic resistance. Science 257:1064–1073

Quintilliani R, Nightingale CH, Crowe HM, Cooper BW, Bartlett RC, Gousse G 1991 Strategic antibiotic decision-making at the formulary level. Rev Infect Dis (suppl 9) 13:770–777

DISCUSSION

Levin: The very impressive decline in frequency of resistance you have shown is really encouraging, but how has this change affected clinical outcomes?

Giamarellou: We are closely following this. So far we haven't been able to attribute any deaths to the control policies.

Summers: Did you see a decrease in infections untreatable by *any* antibiotics? In other words, did the reduction of particular antibiotics spill over into untreatable infections generally? You controlled a couple of specific classes of antibiotics.

Giamarellou: I can't answer that exactly. In trying to check how the hygienic measures have worked in the hospital, we have done many faecal cultures from patients in the vicinity of those who were sick with multiresistant strains. Very rarely did we find that patients in the vicinity were colonized with those multiresistant strains. We put red dots on the charts of patients with a multiresistant strain so that the hospital personnel would be extremely careful handling them.

Baquero: You have told us about Laiko General Hospital: what is the situation in other hospitals in Greece?

Giamarellou: We presented our data at the Ministry of Health, asking for our system to be applied in other hospitals, and it was approved. They started four years ago, but these hospitals do not have infectious disease clinicians, and so although they have tried, the clinical microbiologists have found it difficult to persuade the surgeons in particular and the clinicians in general to implement these measures. I think that the presence of infectious disease clinicians is extremely important for the success of this sort of approach.

Lerner: We have used a similar antibiotic order form for a number of years, but there are situations in which we can't require documentation. We feel there are clinical situations in which suspicion of a role of resistant organisms mandates empiric therapy. For example, what do you do with febrile neutropenic patients who lack an obvious site of infection, or HIV-infected patients who come in with pneumonia which we now recognize may in many cases be due to *Pseudomonas*? You must have a number of built in mechanisms to handle such situations where there isn't the required documentation.

Giamarellou: We reached consensus agreements with the haematologists for febrile neutropenia. If a patient returns to the hospital on several occasions and they get a fever of unknown origin, while waiting for the culture results physicians are always permitted to begin with ceftazidime plus amikacin and to get the approval on the next day. If the patient is a newly introduced case then we would not usually start with the advanced antibiotics. However, if these patients get septic shock, while we are waiting for culture results we always administer vancomycin plus imipenem to cover the possibility of nosocomial multiresistant bacteraemia. Before this system was implemented, all neutropenics were on vancomycin and imipenem from the day they were admitted.

Gaynes: You mentioned you had planned to show your administrators the cost savings your scheme would achieve. Could you comment on this?

Giamarellou: The executive committee is so satisfied with our savings they let us do whatever we want.

Levy: Can you put a figure on the saving? Did you tell them that you had saved them 30–40%, for example?

Giamarellou: It was much more, about 60%, because vancomycin and imipenem are extremely expensive antibiotics.

Gaynes: It seems as if this is a tremendous effort on the part of yourself and the other infectious disease physicians. Is this something that you think you and other hospitals can sustain?

Giamarellou: That's the big question, because after a while one gets tired of all the work this sort of programme entails. Initially it took one-third of my time to organize this system and to check its functioning. However, if you have younger colleagues you can get them to do it and rotate them, and in this way it is not so tiring.

Levy: Pentti Huovinen, you told us that you gave out an educational booklet, and that alone may have changed the attitude of physicians. My understanding is that booklets come and go all the time, but unless you sit down face to face with the prescriber you won't get your message across.

Huovinen: I don't know how effective the books were, but the crucial part of our strategy to reduce erythromycin use was the press release. If you want to catch Finnish doctors, the television news is the most effective means. We have only three national channels, and at least half of the medical doctors are watching the news.

Bennish: Your study suggests that the hospital is an isolated ecosystem, but you're still within the sea of promiscuous use outside the hospital. Often when one tries to implement control measures, especially in developing countries, the hospital can manage it but the community can't. Were your cultures taken from people when they were admitted to hospital? Were they blood, faecal or skin isolates?

Giamarellou: Our recent collections represent blood, pus, urine and sputum isolates of nosocomial origin. Last week our biologists finished the pulse-field gel electrophoresis typing and identified 17 different types of *Pseudomonas aeruginosa* and seven different serotypes among nosocomial multiresistant strains. We have six different *Klebsiellas*, so it's not just the same strain which is circulating. What I realized is that quinolone-resistant strains have been introduced from the community several times, because quinolones can be bought over the counter. I am pessimistic that whatever we do, resistant clones will be introduced from the community.

Levy: The hospital really isn't a totally isolated unit since it is connected with the community. Somehow we have to understand why a change of policy in a hospital can have such a dramatic effect on the bacteria associated with the patients in the hospital, since many of us believe that these organisms — at least some of the Gram-negatives — are brought into the hospital. This brings back the ecology question: is it possible that in the community resistant strains are being selected for by antibiotics, but when they get into hospital they are then under a different selection? They could either be selected against or selected for. If your antibiotic policy prevents transient bacteria from being selected, you will be really providing other (i.e. susceptible) bacteria with a chance.

We've seen a good correlation between antibiotic use and resistance, notably in isolated systems. Now we're struggling with a reversal. Helen has shown us that the reduction of antibiotic use can decrease resistance. How does this happen? Are resistant bacteria really at a selective disadvantage? If the community is constantly receiving antibiotics and the patients are coming from the community, could the hospital be considered a 'cleansing unit' rather than the other way round? It sounds as if I were in Greece I would want to go Laiko General Hospital to get cleaned up! What is going on ecologically?

Lipsitch: These results are often expressed in percentages, but percentage of resistance can go up in one of two ways: either the number of resistant bacteria goes up or the number of susceptible bacteria goes down. One can imagine at least two extremes. In one, susceptible and resistant organisms spread completely independently of each other, so when we see an increase in use it just kills off the susceptibles and the number of resistant bacteria stays the same, but measured as a percentage it looks like it has become worse. In this case it has got better because there are fewer total cases — it is just that most of them are now the resistant ones. The other extreme is that there is competition: there is one habitat, one set of niches, in which these two kinds of bacteria are competing. When you kill off the susceptibles the actual number of resistant bacteria or resistant cases goes up. Is there a way to measure incidence in absolute numbers?

Gaynes: I think one has also to consider another aspect, which I call 'surveillance artifact'. You don't know about resistance unless somebody has ordered a culture, and there is evidence that the culturing frequency of different physicians varies dramatically. In the ICU I have often thought that nurses must feel that getting a culture is somehow therapeutic! It's much less likely that resistance is missed in certain ICUs because patients are always cultured. There's a huge potential for artifact here. This is one of the differences between studying resistance and studying infections. Patients will present with symptoms or signs that are hard to ignore, but you may not know about resistance unless someone has done a culture. Another aspect of the question is estimating the magnitude of resistance in a hospital. One can determine the estimate on the basis of the size of the denominator (the number tested for resistance). Statistical tests can be performed to determine whether one is dealing with significant differences. The size of the denominator can be affected simply by the artifact of the number of cultures.

Lipsitch: Do you find when there is increased use of these antibiotics that the number of total infections changes?

Gaynes: In our system we have generally found that the number tested has not changed dramatically, so I'm assuming that the culture frequency is going to be about the same. We're dealing with big numbers. How this is affected by antibiotic use and whether culturing frequency is related to antibiotic use, I do not know.

Levy: The antibiotic affects the target organism as well as the non-target organisms. It is possible that when antibiotics in the hospital are changed other bacteria will rise or fall secondarily.

Gaynes: Stenotrophomonas maltophilia is intrinsically resistant to an enormous number of antibiotics, notably imipenem, and while that aspect of it hasn't changed for a number of years, it is starting to fill a niche vacated by some of the formerly susceptible pseudomonads and serratias that are normally found in hospitals.

Summers: Ruth Hall has shown that the position of insertion of a given cassette within the integron influences its expressibility. This raises the issue of cryptic genes. In other words, you're looking for expression when you look for phenotype, but the gene may be present and not expressed. A molecular example of this is the integron position, so that if the gene is two or three reading frames downstream from the promoter you could screen for it and not see it because its expression will be very low. A few rearrangements of that integron later on and that same gene could be right next to the promoter and now you've got an expressed resistance. Just because you don't see the phenotype expressed, this doesn't mean the gene is not present in the strain.

Bennish: I wanted to get back to the issue of what constitutes an ecological unit. The direct correlate between antimicrobial use and resistance breaks down a bit if you look on a global scale for certain community-acquired pathogens. If you look at pneumococcus, gonococcus and the enteric pathogens, resistance arose first in developing countries where the absolute magnitude of antibiotic use is logs lower than in western countries. Pneumococcal resistance developed in New Guinea, *Shigella* multiple resistance has recently developed in areas where *Shigella* was endemic (Central Africa and Southern Asia), *Salmonella* Typhi multiple resistance developed in South Asia, and cholera resistance has developed in many countries. These are all areas where the majority of infections go untreated. For example, in Bangladesh *Shigella dysenteriae* type I resistance to co-trimoxazule went from 5% to 80% within two years.

Spratt: The Papua New Guinea pneumococcal story is probably explained by the massive use of penicillin to control Yaws.

Bennish: In some ways that reinforces my point, in that these are very special ecological considerations, so the attempt to make a direct correlate with antibiotic use in the development of resistance breaks down, at least in the organisms that I'm familiar with.

Davies: Shigella dysentery was epidemic in Japan after the war, and enormous amounts of antibiotics were introduced into an (essentially) antibiotic virgin community. Levels of resistance to these antibiotics in *Shigella* spp. increased rapidly — that's where multiple resistance was first found.

Levin: By increasing the density of the bacteria you are also increasing the rate of infectious transfer of the plasmids. Thus, part of the ascent of the resistance plasmid may be accounted for by transfer as well as selection.

Davies: I don't think this is the point; I'm saying that antibiotic resistance in the bacterial population arises as the direct result of extensive antibiotic use; Mike Bennish is saying it is not happening.

Bennish: I'm not saying that selective pressure does not happen. I'm just saying that in terms of modelling, the magnitude of antimicrobial use might not be the critical factor, at least for pathogens as contrasted with nosocomial flora. Rather, what I am asking is how selective pressure exerts itself within different communities. Even with what we think is controlled use we can see the development of widespread resistance.

Cohen: One has to think of the frequency of resistance as having two major components. The first is the influence of antibiotic use, and the second is the transmission of resistant organisms. In all these geographic areas you're describing, there are high levels of transmission, so perhaps one needs fewer genetic events to occur for resistance to emerge.

Bennish: The point is, in areas of intense transmission the models that you're postulating for control might be much less effective than experience in other settings suggests.

Gaynes: That's one of the ideas behind what I was presenting: even in places where you assume that antibiotic use is the big issue, for example an ICU, there's still wide variation between different ICUs. Consequently, one can't always show a relationship between use and resistance. This is where cross-transmission is probably occurring. Yet, if you just knew the resistance level in a certain ICU without knowing its antibiotic use, you couldn't make any interpretation as to which was happening more. In the developing world cross-transmission probably dominates, so this issue is probably also relevant there.

Witte: When we look at developing countries, we shouldn't forget about inappropriate use of antibiotics. Before the fall of the 'iron curtain' we got information from Mongolia, Vietnam, Angola and Ethiopia about the appearance of multiresistant staphylococci outside hospitals. We got a lot of information on the inappropriate use of antibiotics, for instance oxicillin against *Salmonella* Typhi in Mongolia.

Huovinen: It is impossible to get any consumption figures from most of these countries. For instance, in several large countries there may be hundreds of different manufacturers of antimicrobial agents.

Bennish: There are two ways to get these figures. Countries such as Bangladesh and the Philippines only import drugs: there's no manufacturer of basic agents in most of these countries, they just package them, so one can look at import figures. It is also possible to do village studies by looking at the number of prescriptions given. Outside urban areas, there is often very little antimicrobial use.

Huovinen: These sorts of consumption data should be collected world-wide.

Copeland: It's very difficult to get these data. Whenever people talk about consumption of antibiotics, the data are kept largely in financial terms. When you actually look at the kilogram usage world-wide, you get a reversal, so that cephalosporins, which by value sell twice as much world-wide as say penicillins, are used half as much by weight. However, it is a myth to think that the Third World accounts for most of the use, because 85% of the world's kilogram usage of antibiotics is probably used by 20–25% of the world's population.

Baquero: There are two further concepts that we ought to address. First, we should consider classifying antibiotics according to their selective power for certain mechanisms of resistance. In Laiko General hospital, it seems that ceftazidime was a huge selector of resistance, and once it was removed, a healthier microbial ecology was recovered. If you have a different type of mechanism of resistance to given bugs, use of selective antibiotics should be reduced to a different level. The second concept for consideration is: is there a threshold level of antibiotic that is selective? If the amount of antibiotic is below a certain level, perhaps the selective activity is low. If the use of antibiotic is increased even a small amount over the threshold level, this might drastically increase the selective process.

Levy: I agree. If you think of this concept in terms of the commensal susceptible strains out there, the threshold is really that level at which you have greatly decreased the potential for susceptible strains to return because you've given such an advantage to the resistant strains.

Gaynes: One thing I have found in hospitals is that for all of the work that you do to decrease antibiotic use, people from pharmaceutical companies come at your physicians doing the exact opposite, trying to increase antibiotic use. Often their salary or commission is dependent on how much your hospital spends on antibiotics.

Bush: As a representative of the pharmaceutical industry I think I might be able to say something the rest of you may be thinking. As a scientist I have been distressed by some of the marketing strategies used to promote inappropriate use of antimicrobial agents. I have seen some instances where the sales force is told that they don't need to understand how a drug works, they just have to sell as much as possible. In contrast, some pharmaceutical companies have tried carefully to educate their marketing people so that they will advocate the appropriate use of an antibiotic. I challenge the pharmaceutical industry to do a better job of education, so that sales personnel will not be advocating the misuse of antimicrobials. There certainly are times when antimicrobial agents should be used, but at these times they should be used appropriately.

Cohen: I'm interested in the behaviour of both the pharmaceutical representatives and the physicians after you imposed your order forms. First, how did the pharmaceutical representatives try to market their drugs in the face of a situation where use had to be justified? Did they actually try to educate the physicians to use the drug appropriately? Second, since you removed so many of those drugs and since it appeared that the physicians were prescribing whatever drug had recently been marketed, what did they actually start using when they couldn't use the controlled pharmaceutical agents?

Giamarellou: When we started our audit system I asked the physicians if they knew which generation of cephalosporins cefazoline belongs to. They thought it was a fourth generation cephalosporin! After applying the restriction policy programme they started using first and second generation cephalosporins, and inhibitors as well. I don't think that we had problems in that respect. The problem was mainly the pharmaceutical representatives who were pushing the physicians to prescribe and to liberate the restricted antibiotics. We tried to explain that it is also in the interests of the drug company for the antibiotics to last. When the physicians realized we were dealing with 50% resistance to ceftazidime, they shifted to imipenem for the critically ill patients with nosocomial sepsis. Glaxo and Eli-Lilly were not happy with this because they both manufacture ceftazidime. It is necessary to be very patient with the drug representatives and we have to explain the situation to them. When we started the programme in 1989, one could even buy imipenem over the counter in Greece. We applied to the Ministry of Health and finally we succeeded in convincing them to make these newer compounds available only in the hospital.

Baquero: We spoke this morning about the environmental health impact of antibiotics. Increasingly, the pharmaceutical industry should consider itself as a pollutant industry that is altering the normal environment on Earth by the impact of antibiotics on the microbial environment. So, in common with other industries, the pharmaceutical industry should have policies to minimize their environmental impact. This philosophy would help a lot in our goal of preventing antibiotic resistance.

Levy: We have come to a new point in antimicrobial understanding—the realization of the environmental and ecological consequences of antibiotics. Moreover, we are witnessing a time when resistant bacteria have emerged to render many antibiotics ineffective and we are searching for new ones.

The antibiotic selective process: concentration-specific amplification of low-level resistant populations

F. Baquero, M. C. Negri, M. I. Morosini and J. Blázquez

Department of Microbiology, Ramón y Cajal Hospital, National Institute of Health (INSALUD), 28034 Madrid, Spain

Abstract. The biochemistry and genetics of antibiotic resistance are far better known than the equally important events underlying the selection of resistant populations. The hidden selection of low-level resistant variants may be a key process in the emergence of high-level antibiotic resistance. Different low-level resistant bacterial subpopulations may be specifically selected by different low antibiotic concentrations. The space in the environment (human body) where a given selective concentration exists represents the selective compartment. For pharmacokinetic reasons, low antibiotic concentrations occur in a larger selective compartment and persist longer than high antibiotic concentrations. The specific selection of low-level variants by low concentrations of antibiotic can be reproduced in experimental *in vitro* models using mixtures of susceptible and low-level resistant populations. We demonstrated this in *Escherichia coli* strains harbouring TEM-1, TEM-12 and TEM-10 β-lactamases challenged by cefotaxime, and also *Streptococcus pneumoniae* strains with various levels of penicillin resistance challenged by amoxicillin or cefotaxime. In both cases, four hours of antibiotic challenge produced selective peaks of low-level resistant variant populations at low-level antibiotic concentrations. We conclude that variants with small decreases in antibiotic susceptibility may be fully selectable under *in vivo* circumstances; on the other hand, low-level antibiotic concentrations may have a considerable selective effect on the emergence of antibiotic resistance.

1997 Antibiotic resistance: origins, evolution, selection and spread. Wiley, Chichester (Ciba Foundation Symposium 207) p 93–111

The development of antibiotic resistance is among the best documented examples we have of contemporary evolution (Shapiro 1992). Currently, impressive advances in understanding the molecular biology of antibiotic resistance contrast with general ignorance of the population ecology of resistant microorganisms. The biochemistry and genetics of antibiotic resistance in individual bacterial cells are far better known than the equally important events explaining the selection of resistant populations. Certainly, most available data support the concept that the use of antibiotics is related to the selection of antibiotic resistant bacteria (Levy 1992, Levy et al 1987,

Tenover & McGowan 1996). Nevertheless, the biological rules of the selective process remain largely unconsidered. Formal studies on population genetics of antibiotic resistance have been recently proposed (Levin et al 1997). Research in this field is urgently needed; such research should be based on a previous theoretical and technological reconsideration of the selective effects of the antibiotics on bacterial populations. This paper discusses some new paradigms and techniques with which we can approach this work.

Low antibiotic concentrations

The current mainstream concepts on the evolution of antibiotic resistance in microorganisms have been dominated by some a priori assumptions. The first of these probably originated from human chemotherapy: to be considered 'resistant' to an antibiotic, a given microorganism must express a relevant increase in the minimum inhibitory concentration (MIC) to this drug. In this view, 'minor' increases are meaningless, since the patient can still be succesfully treated with antibiotic concentrations exceeding this MIC value (the 'blood' level is generally considered). The second assumption, derived from the first, is that 'only significant antibiotic concentrations apply in selection of resistance'. Therefore, as antibiotics are mostly excreted in very small amounts by natural microorganisms in the environment, the origin of resistance as a result of these small selective forces, outside of the producing organism (Davies 1992), tends to be disregarded. A third assumption, also closely related to the first, is that 'resistance genes' are only those genes related to 'significant' high-level resistance. The main purpose of this paper is to stress the selective importance of low antibiotic concentrations. Under natural circumstances, the preservation of susceptible bacteria may depend on the fact that the selective effect could be preferentially exerted in a given spatial compartment-in a 'small niche' according to Maynard Smith & Hoekstra (1980). We propose that this selective compartment, responsible for this type of 'confined selection', could be considered to be the virtual space or niche in which a precise concentration of antibiotic provides a specific selection of a particular resistant bacterial variant. The antibiotic concentration exerting such an effect is here designated as the 'selective antibiotic concentration'.

Concentration-specific selection

Antibiotics used in chemotherapy create large concentration gradients. These gradients are due to pharmacokinetic factors, such as the different diffusion rates into various tissues, metabolism, local inactivation, or variation in the elimination rate from different compartments. The direct effect of microbes of the normal or pathogenic flora, particularly (but not exclusively) if they possess antibiotic-inactivating enzymes, also contributes to gradient formation. In general, high antibiotic concentrations will be confined to small and ephemeral selective compartments, and low concentrations are expected to be distributed over longer times in larger selective compartments. Most bacterial populations in the human microflora probably face a wide range of antibiotic concentrations after each administration of the drug. Since the spontaneous genetic variability of microbial populations also provides a wide range of potentially selectable subpopulations, it is appropriate to determine which antibiotic concentration is able to select one or other of these particular subpopulations.

Any antibiotic concentration has the potential to select a resistant variant if it is able to inhibit growth of the susceptible population but not that of the variant harbouring the resistance mechanism. In other words, a selective antibiotic concentration is that which exceeds the MIC (under the local conditions) of the more susceptible population, but not that of the variant population (even if it is very close). If MICs of both susceptible and variant populations are surpassed, then no selection of the variant will occur; the same applies when the antibiotic concentration is below the local MICs of both populations. Therefore, the selection of a particular variant happens only in a narrow range of drug concentrations (Baquero et al 1993). The principle behind this type of concentration-specific selection is illustrated in Fig. 1.

Theoretically, each particular variant population showing a definite MIC will have the possibility of being selectively enriched by a particular antibiotic concentration. This conclusion appears obvious. Surprisingly, the theoretical and practical consequences of such a conclusion remain to be explored.

Selective amplification of β-lactamase molecular variants

TEM-1 β-lactamase is considered to be a broad-spectrum enzyme because it hydrolyses both penicillins and cephalosporins. However, it cannot efficiently inactivate new extended-spectrum cephalosporins and monobactam agents, such as cefotaxime, ceftazidime or aztreonam. Molecular variants of TEM-1 (or TEM-2, which differs only in one amino acid), have acquired the ability to hydrolyse such substrates. These variants, termed extended-spectrum β-lactamases (ESBLs), emerged and disseminated probably as a consequence of the introduction of these extended-spectrum β-lactam antibiotics into the therapeutic armamentarium. In some cases, antibiotic-inactivating ESBLs differ from TEM-1 by only two to five amino acid substitutions. For instance, TEM-10 differs from TEM-1 in the Arg164Ser and Glu240Lys substitutions, which increase the cefotaxime MIC from 0.03 to 1 μg/ml. It seems obvious that enzymes like TEM-10 should have evolved under cefotaxime selection from previous TEM-1 variants with a single amino acid substitution: for instance, TEM-12 (with only the Arg164 replacement) is a likely ancestor of TEM-10. This implies that strains harbouring TEM-10, despite the very low increase in the MIC of certain extended spectrum cephalosporins (0.06–0.12 μg/ml for cefotaxime, compared with 0.03 μg/ml for TEM-1), were indeed selected during therapy, and enriched to a sufficient extent to increase the possibility of the development of another point mutation leading to a more effective resistance. Bacteria carrying TEM-12 and most

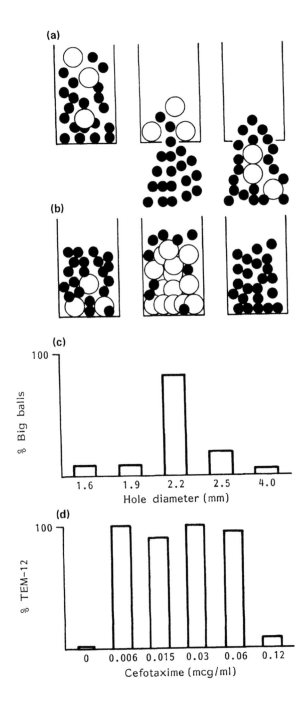

(a)

(b)

(c)

100 —

% Big balls

1.6   1.9   2.2   2.5   4.0

Hole diameter (mm)

(d)

100 —

% TEM-12

0   0.006 0.015   0.03   0.06   0.12

Cefotaxime (mcg/ml)

other single-amino-acid replaced TEM β-lactamases are rarely detected in clinical microbiology laboratories: they are too similar in terms of susceptibility to those having the classical TEM-1! Nevertheless, the epidemiology of clinical resistance to extended-spectrum cephalosporins may depend on the detection of such early mutants and the consequent adjustment of specific policies of antibiotic use in a particular community.

In order to test this model of selective antibiotic concentrations, we studied the selective amplification by cefotaxime of bacterial populations containing TEM-12 over TEM-1, and TEM10 over TEM-12 and TEM-1, in mixed cultures. Isogenic bacteria, differing only in a single amino acid replacement in the β-lactamase enyme (Blázquez et al 1995), were used to mimic the mutational variation from a single original clone. *Escherichia coli* MC4100:K-*12* F$^-$ *araD139 (argF-lac)U169 flbB5301 fruA25 relA1 rpsL150 rbsR* (Casadaban 1976), and nalidixic-resistant (Nal^r) and spectinomycin-resistant (Spc^r) derivatives were used at host strains. pBGTEM-1 was constructed by cloning a *Bam*HI-*Bam*HI fragment from the plasmid pKT254Δ-Ap (Fellay et al 1987) containing the *bla*T1 (TEM-1 β-lactamase) gene from Tn*3* into the *Bam*HI site of the non-conjugative plasmid pBGS19$^-$. The Arg164Ser (pBGTEM-12) and Arg164Ser plus Glu240Lys (pBGTEM-10) mutants were constructed by site-directed mutagenesis (Kunkel 1987). The plasmids pBGTEM-12 and pBGTEM-10 were introduced into the Nal^r and Spc^r MC4100 variants; the plasmid pBGTEM-1 was in the MC4100 wild strain. The MICs of these MC4100 derivatives to cefotaxime were 0.03 μg/ml (for strains containing TEM-1), 0.06 μg/ml (TEM-12) and 1 μg/ml (TEM-10). The five MC4100 derivatives were grown overnight in Mueller–Hinton broth, reaching 2×10^8 cfu/ml. The proportions of the mixture tended to reflect the predominance of the wild TEM-1 harbouring population, with a lesser representation of the single mutant TEM-12 population (10%) and even lower proportion of the double TEM-10 mutant (1%). One millilitre of each mixture (total count, 2×10^5 cfu/ml) was used to inoculate an equivalent volume of brain heart infusion broth tubes containing different cefotaxime concentrations, and control

FIG. 1. (*opposite*) Elementary representation of the principle of concentration-specific selection. Small balls (sensitive, S) represent a biological subpopulation susceptible to low concentrations of an inhibitor; large (resistant, R) balls represent another subpopulation requiring higher concentrations for inhibition. The size of the hole in the bottom of the boxes represents the concentration of the inhibitor. (a) The effect of piercing holes of two different sizes: if the hole is very small (left), no balls are eliminated; when the size the hole exceeds a critical size, only S balls are dropping (centre); at a wider diameter, both S and R balls drop (right). (b) The holes were closed after a certain time, and the S or R balls remaining into the boxes at this moment ('surviving balls') multiply at the same rate until the original population was reached again. Note the selection (predominance) of the R balls at a particular hole size (centre), but not in the lower (left) or higher (right) sizes. (c) Results obtained in a mechanical model with real steel balls. (d) Results of a experimental *in vitro* selection of *Escherichia coli* cells containing TEM-12 β-lactamase (R) over TEM-1 (S) at various cefotaxime concentrations (see text for details).

tubes without antibiotic. All tubes were then incubated for 4 h at 37 °C, to reflect the expected period of contact of bacterial populations with such a range of concentrations in the human body. After this challenge, the survivor cells of the original populations were allowed to grow overnight in a fresh, antibiotic-free medium (containing β-lactamase type IV from *Enterobacter cloacae*) to allow subsequent amplification of the populations selected during the period of exposure to the antibiotic. This amplification period may imitate the expected recolonization process after chemotherapy. In fact, most of the epidemiological consequences of the selection of resistant variants are dependent upon the metapopulation resulting from this late regrowth phase. Then, individual colonies were obtained in Columbia agar, and further identified in selective plates to calculate the change in final proportions of the different bacterial populations originally seeded.

As summarized in Fig. 2 (upper part), in the culture containing a very low cefotaxime concentration (0.008 μg/ml), TEM-12 was clearly selected, and the predominance of the TEM-12-containing population in subculture was maintained at 0.015, 0.03 and 0.06 μg/ml. Maximal selection of TEM-12 over TEM-1 was reached in the interval of concentrations ranging from 0.008 to 0.06 μg/ml. This was considered to be the TEM-12 interval of cefotaxime selective concentrations under the assay conditions. As expected from the selective amplification concept, above these concentrations, at only 0.12 μg/ml, the strong selection of TEM-12 disappeared and TEM-1 remained dominant. At this concentration, TEM-1 and TEM-12 were *both* counterselected and, therefore, the originally predominant TEM-1 population (even if its absolute number was decreased) remained predominant among the survivor cells and therefore accounted for the highest proportion of cells in the subsequent antibiotic-free culture.

In triple cultures (Fig. 2, bottom) the selective amplification of TEM-12 over TEM-1 described above was repeated at a similar range to that in the previous experiments, 0.008–0.03 μg/ml. Obviously, TEM-10 should have been co-selected with TEM-12 over TEM-1 with this range of concentration, but considering its original minor proportion in relation to TEM-12, most survivor cells contained TEM-12 and this population maintained its predominance over TEM-10 after subculture amplification. As in the double culture experiment, TEM-1 remained the predominant population in cultures challenged with the next concentration, in this case 0.06 μg/ml. At this concentration, TEM-12 was not selected and the TEM-1-containing population (even if its absolute number was decreased), remained sufficient to predominate in subcultures over the TEM-10 population. In cultures challenged with 0.12 μg/ml cefotaxime, TEM-1-containing cells suddenly emerged in subcultures and constituted the predominant population, clearly because of the selective inhibition of TEM-1 and TEM-12 variant populations (Fig. 3). Essentially the same results were obtained regardless of which population carried the Nal^R or the Spc^R marker. Mathematical modelling of the effect of selective antibiotic concentrations on mixed bacterial populations is possible and reproduces the experimental results (M. C. Negri, M. Lipsitch, B. R. Levin & F. Baquero, unpublished results).

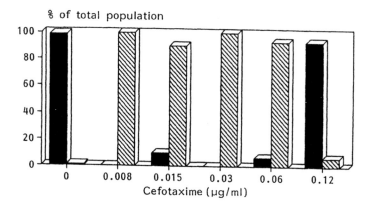

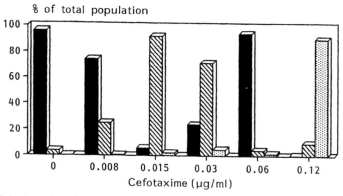

FIG. 2.   Selective cefotaxime concentrations for TEM-1 β-lactamase mutant strains containing TEM-12, with a single amino acid substitution (Arg164Ser), increasing cefotaxime MIC from 0.03 (TEM-1) to 0.12 μg/ml, and TEM-10, with two substitutions (Arg164Ser, Glu240Lys) which increases the MIC to 1 μg/ml. Upper part, mixed inoculum with TEM-1 (90%, black bars), and TEM-12 (10%, hatched bars). Lower part, mixed inoculum containing all three strains at the proportions 89% (TEM-1), 10% (TEM-12) and 1% (TEM-10, stippled bars). Inocula were seeded on tubes containing different cefotaxime concentrations, and a control tube without antibiotic. After 4 h, the antibiotic was enzymically removed, the survivors were allowed to grow overnight in fresh drug-free medium, and the culture was plated for colony analysis. Bars represent the final proportion of TEM-1, TEM-12 and TEM-10 harbouring strains in each tube as determined after the study of 100–200 colonies (mean value of three separate experiments).

Selective amplification of penicillin-resistant
Streptococcus pneumoniae populations

At the epidemiological level, the natural history of the development of *S. pneumoniae* resistance in different countries (Baquero 1996) supports the concept that the early selection of low-level resistant variants generally precedes the emergence of

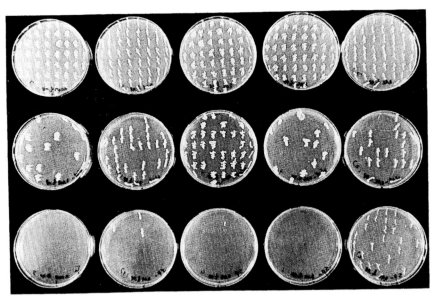

FIG. 3.   The selective concentration as it is appreciated in a typical experiment using conditions similar to those of Fig. 2 (lower part). Upper row, colonies in non-selective medium (TEM-1+TEM-12+TEM-10). Middle row, colonies in selective medium for TEM-12; lower row, selective medium for TEM-10. Colonies seeded in the first column (left) are in provenance from mixed cultures challenged by very low cefotaxime concentrations; from left to right, concentrations are growing. Note that TEM-12 (middle row) is preferentially selected at intermediate concentrations, and TEM-10 (bottom row), at high concentrations.

high-level resistance (Fig. 4). We have recently proposed a model of antibiotic-selective amplification to explain the development of penicillin resistance in *S. pneumoniae* (Negri et al 1994). In this case, the selective pressure after 4 h of exposure to different concentrations of β-lactam agents was evaluated in a mixture of *S. pneumoniae* populations with low or high-level penicillin resistance. The proportion in the original culture of susceptible : intermediate : resistant strains was 90 : 9 : 1. As in the case of TEM β-lactamase, at a particular range of concentrations of each of the different antibiotics (selectors) used, a particular strain with a given penicillin MIC was selected. For instance, at the extremely low amoxycillin concentration of 0.015 μg/ml, the strain with intermediate MIC to penicillin was strongly selected against the predominant penicillin-susceptible strain (Fig. 5). Nevertheless, at 2 μg/ml, most of the survivor cells corresponded to the originally predominant susceptible population and, therefore, the intermediate resistant strain was much less efficiently selected. In the case of cefotaxime, the intermediate penicillin-resistant strain had its selection peak at 0.015 mg/ml of cefotaxime and the more resistant one at 0.25 μg/ml, the more susceptible strain predominating at 0.5 and 1 μg/ml. This example illustrates once

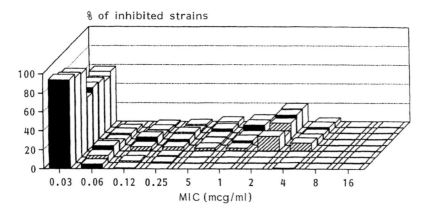

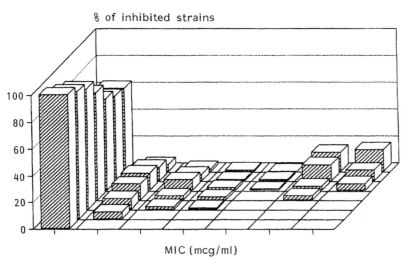

FIG. 4. (*Top*) Distribution of *Streptococcus pneumoniae* isolates accordingly to their penicillin MICs in different European towns and periods. From the front to the rear, London 1992, London 1993, Paris 1992, Paris 1993, Toulouse 1992, Toulouse 1993, Barcelona 1992 and Barcelona 1993. Data from the Alexander Project (Baquero 1996). (*Bottom*) A presumptive model of the expected evolution of penicillin resistance in *S. pneumoniae* inspired by these data.

again the selective amplification of bacterial populations at particular antibiotic concentrations.

Antibiotic concentration-specific selection: evolutionary implications

In summary, these experiments show that the emergence by selection of some antibiotic-resistant bacterial populations (including low-level mutants) may occur

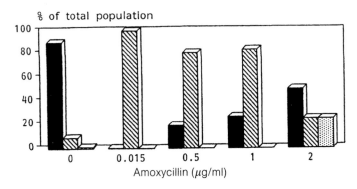

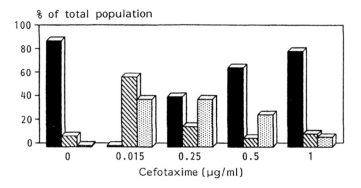

FIG. 5. Selective amoxycillin and cefotaxime concentrations for *Streptococcus pneumoniae* RYC28057 strains with low-level resistance to penicillin (MIC 0.5 μg/ml), and RYC28543 and RYC099X2 strains with high-level resistance (MICs 1 μg/ml and 2 μg/ml, respectively). The strain RYC28551 with a penicillin MIC of 0.015 μg/ml was considered to be fully susceptible. A mixed inoculum containing all four strains at the proportions 90% (RYC28551), 9% (RYC28057) and 1% (RYC28543 plus RYC09982) was seeded on tubes containing different amoxycillin concentrations. After four hours, the antibiotic was enzymically removed and the survivor cells were allowed to grow overnight in fresh drug-free medium tubes, and then culture was plated for colony analysis. Bars represent the final proportion of penicillin susceptible (black bars), low-level (hatched bars) and high-level resistant strains (pointed bars) as determined after the study of about 50 colonies (mean value of three separate experiments).

only at certain antibiotic concentrations — the 'selective antibiotic concentrations' for such a population under the conditions of the challenge. In our experimental examples, these elementary conditions included planctonic type of growth, absolute predominance in numbers of the more susceptible strains, and a single 'round' of antibiotic challenge. Even considering the limitations of the study, some general points for discussion inspired by the observed phenomena could be proposed.

(1) The adaptive value of minor phenotypic changes

An extremely small increase in MIC seemed to be sufficient to give an important increase in selection, provided adequate conditions were present. This conclusion seems to contradict the widespread opinion that if the phenotypic effect of a mutation is very low, its contribution to a selective advantage in fitness for the species should be similarly low (Kimura 1983, Hartl et al 1985). The evolutionary significance of some recently isolated TEM-1 mutants showing very small increases in MIC was considered obscure by the authors 'since we do not know how small an effect constitutes a selective advantage' (Huang et al 1994). In fact, our data suggest that the fate of a given mutation may depend on the possibility of a successful encounter of the mutant organism with its particular selective concentration.

(2) The selective value of minor environmental changes

The re-evaluation of the possibility of important ecological effects produced by very small concentrations of antibiotics released to the environment may be of interest. For instance, the natural biological effect of antibiotics-and probably of most secondary metabolites — may not be understood if these potential effects on closely located microbial populations are disregarded. 'The genes and the enzymes (for secondary metabolites) are there, but they are not very functional! I don't know the significance of this, but it's often overlooked' said J. D. Bu'Lock in the discussion of a Cavalier-Smith (1992) paper. Our opinion is that they *are* frequently functional, but not under the particular conditions fixed by the observer. Very small concentrations of the agent could exert an unexpected, strong biological effect on the relative proportions within adequately chosen mixtures of responder and non-responder bacteria. This approach could eventually be applicable to the re-evaluation of the potential for development of antibiotic resistance among bacteria surrounding antibiotic-producing organisms. According to our data, even the very low antibiotic concentrations attainable by diffussion in the vicinity of these organisms could be sufficient to select bacteria harbouring mechanisms of resistance. The same type of reasoning could be applied to the evaluation of the potential selective effects of small concentrations of antibiotics present in foodstuffs as a result of antibiotic-supplemented feed used to enhance animal growth.

(3) Bacterial genetic diversity and variability in concentration gradients

Bacterial populations show impressive natural genetic polymorphism. For many antibiotics, spontaneous gene variation frequently results in a multiplicity of low-level mechanisms of resistance, the emergence of more specific high-level mechanisms being less frequent (except for a limited number of antibiotics, or by the uptake of exogenous highly specialized genes). In the real world, antibiotic concentrations challenging bacteria are mostly relatively low (large selective compartment), and those populations showing small increases in MIC would be expected to be preferentially selected by these antibiotics. We should insist once more on the importance of the selection of low-level resistant bacterial mutants to explain the spread of high-level resistance. First of all, several consecutive rounds of selection at the selective antibiotic concentration will produce a progressive enrichment of the low-level variant, and this occurs during most multi-dose treatments (Moreillon & Tomasz 1988). Once a critical number is reached, new variants may arise, which can now be selected in the following selective antibiotic concentration, so increasing the antibiotic resistance level. On the other hand, low-level resistant variants can reach a 'survival' position permitting the incorporation of foreign resistance genes in an antibiotic-rich medium.

In conclusion, these studies of population-selective amplification suggest that at different points of a concentration gradient, selective forces may be acting with different selective specificity. To a certain extent, the continuous variation of antibiotic concentrations may resemble a tuning device which selects a certain radio frequency. Under or over such a frequency (the antibiotic selective concentration), the emission (the particular variant) is lost (selection does not take place). The saddle between the concentrations inhibiting the susceptible and resistant populations is the frequency signal recognized by the selective concentration. Obviously, if any selective factor is made up of a very large number of individual specific selective forces acting in compartmentalized areas, the field for potential selection of variants will be enormously enlarged, which permits a better understanding of the observed overwhelming microbial genetic diversity. In a sense, every quantity in a given gradient can be conceived now as a quality with a distinctive selective potential for a particular mutant.

Gottfried Wilhelm Leibniz, the person who contributed most both in philosophy and mathematics to the understanding of a *continuum* as composed of a multiplicity of qualitatively different units of activity, visited Antony van Leeuwenhoek at his home at Delft in 1676. The time has come for microbiologists to return this visit to Leibniz and to discuss with him the applications of the basic concepts which permitted the discovery of *Calculi Differentialis*, to the elucidation of the clues of microbial evolution.

Acknowledgements

This work is dedicated to Professor Yves-Achille Chabbert, who first introduced one of us (F. B.) to the field of the ecology of bacterial resistance to antibiotics. Concerning the hypothesis discussed in this paper, the authors received encouragement and suggestions from R. Antia, F. J. Ayala, P. Courvalin, J. Davies, J. M. Gómez-Gomez, D. Hopwood, C. Kunin, B. Levin, R. Lenski, S. Levy, M. Lipsitch, A. Medeiros, H. Neu, I. Phillips, M. Schaechter, C. Sanders and D. Shlaes.

References

Baquero F 1996 Trends in antibiotic resistance of respiratory pathogens: an analysis and commentary on a collaborative surveillance study. J Antimicrob Chemother 38:117–132

Baquero F, Negri MC, Morosini MI, Blázquez J 1993 Effect of selective antibiotic concentrations on the evolution of antimicrobial resistance. APUA Newsletter 11:4–5

Blázquez J, Morosini MI, Negri MC, Gonzalez-Leiza M, Baquero F 1995 Single amino acid replacements in positions altered in naturally occurring extended-spectrum TEM β-lactamases. Antimicrob Agents Chemother 39:145–149

Cavalier-Smith T 1992 Origins of secondary metabolism. In: Secondary metabolites: their function and evolution. Wiley, Chichester (Ciba Found Symp 171) p 64–87

Davies J 1992 Another look at antibiotic resistance. J Gen Microbiol 138:1553–1559

Fellay RJ, Frey J, Kirsch H 1987 Interposon mutagenesis of soil and water bacteria: a family of DNA fragments designed for in vitro insertional mutagenesis of Gram-negative bacteria. Gene 52:147–154

Hartl DL, Dykhuizen DE, Dean AM 1985 Limits of adaptation: the evolution of selective neutrality. Genetics 111:655–674

Huang, W, Quyen-Quyen L, LaRocco M, Palzkill T 1994 Effect of threonine-to-methionine substitution at position 265 on structure and function of TEM-1 β-lactamase. Antimicrob Agents Chemother 38:2266–2269

Kimura M 1983 The neutral theory of molecular evolution. Cambridge University Press, Cambridge

Kunkel TA 1987 Rapid and efficient site-specific mutagenesis without phenotypic selection. Methods Enzymol 154:367–382

Levin BR, Lipsitch M, Perrot V et al 1997 The population genetics of antibiotic resistance. Clin Infect Dis, in press

Levy SB 1992 The antibiotic paradox: how miracle drugs are destroying the miracle. Plenum, New York

Levy SB, Burke JP, Wallace CK (eds) 1987 Antibiotic use and antibiotic resistance worldwide. Rev Infect Dis (suppl 3) 9

Maynard-Smith J, Hoekstra R 1980 Polymorphism in a varied environment: how robust are the models? Genet Res Camb 35:45–57

Moreillon P, Tomasz A 1988 Penicillin resistance and defective lysis in clinical isolates of pneumococci: evidence for two kinds of antibiotic pressure operating in the clinical environment. J Infect Dis 157:1150–1157

Negri MC, Morosini MI, Loza E, Baquero F 1994 In vitro selective antibiotic concentrations of β-lactams for penicillin-resistant Streptococcus pneumoniae populations. Antimicrob Agents Chemother 38:122–125

Shapiro JA 1992 Natural genetic engineering in evolution. Genetica 86:99–111

Tenover FC, McGowan JE 1996 Reasons for the emergence of antibiotic resistance. Am J Med Sci 311:9–16

DISCUSSION

Summers: If I understand you correctly, then any kind of an antibiotic dose, even a very strong one, will inevitably result in a pulse of diluted low-level antibiotic in the body. In other words, this effect is unavoidable when antibiotic is given.

Baquero: That is true. It can only be avoided if you are giving very small antibiotic concentrations, in which case there will be compartments with such low antibiotic concentrations that there will be no cidal activity. For low antibiotic dosages compartments may exist without antibiotic, but obviously if the dose is increased, all compartments would be to a certain extent under selection of the antibiotic.

Summers: Do you presently view this model as applying primarily to conventional point mutation-type changes?

Baquero: Corpet et al (1989) demonstrated in a gnotobiotic animal model that very low antibiotic concentrations present in the gut from oral therapy were able to select, at low antibiotic concentrations, some plasmid-mediated resistant populations.

Nowak: It is interesting that your model proposes no selection at high drug concentrations. Is this only found in specific systems or is this a general observation? If so, what are the practical implications?

Baquero: I am not able to generalize. We have been trying to reproduce the structure of populations using a susceptible to mutant ratio of 100:1. This is probably not realistic — the real proportion may well be closer to a million to one. If we were to adapt our set-up to include a huge predominance of the susceptible strains we could probably adapt our model to be more like the real-life situation. On the other hand, the model presented here considers that the MIC of the mutant is close to that of the wild strain.

Nowak: But is the general belief in the antibiotic world that if the concentration is high enough any mutations will be suppressed?

Baquero: Yes. At relatively high antibiotic concentrations the selection of the mutant is suppressed, as the statistical possibility of survival (for the same killing rate) is higher for the susceptible population, but outnumbers the resistant one.

Miller: However, there will always be compartments where the concentration is lower, and there will always be a lower concentration at the end of therapy.

Bennish: I want to apply this model to the real-life hospital intensive care unit (ICU) situation as described by Robert Gaynes in his paper (Gaynes & Monnet 1997, this volume), where he implied that perhaps only 10% of the acquisition of resistance in ICUs is through cross-transmission. Is the remaining 90% accounted for by people who come in with low level resistant mutants, small populations of which are not detected and are then selected for?

Gaynes: The work that Bob Weinstein did a number of years ago looking at aminoglycoside resistance tends to support this, particularly in *Pseudomonas* (Weinstein et al 1980). The dominant mechanism of *Pseudomonas* aminoglycoside resistance is by the blocking of uptake. This stems from mutations in the chromosome rather than an acquired resistance based on plasmid-borne modifying enzymes. Bob showed clinically that barrier precautions stringently applied can prevent acquired resistance, i.e. cross-transmission, but that the antibiotic use paralleled the isolation of the resistant *Pseudomonas*. This suggests that mutation is occurring or that selection is occurring for a resistant subpopulation. He's extended that work to look at patients that have come into the ICU, culturing them for resistant subpopulations, and has found that an amazing number of patients admitted to the ICU who have absolutely no history of antibiotic use, nor any history of exposure to individuals who have been in the hospital, have these resistant subpopulations.

Baquero: A more generalized view of what has been presented here was mentioned by Stuart Levy yesterday. Imagine that there are different mechanisms of resistance that are not very successful against high antibiotic concentrations but are still sufficient to decrease the killing rate of the drugs. These might serve as a first step in the acquisition of more effective mechanisms of resistance by keeping the bacteria alive at a level sufficient for them to be able to accept plasmids bearing resistance determinants from donor microorganisms.

Levy: I want to clarify a point. When we look at the MIC (minimum inhibitory concentration) we are observing the inhibition of growth. In fact, our studies suggest that a small increase in the MIC can cause a big change in the MBC (minimum bactericidal concentration). Dead bacteria don't become resistant! If, for example, a small TEM-1 mutation only increases the MIC a little but changes the MBC a lot, the consequence is larger than the small increase in MIC. The cells are not dead — while they are not growing they are still subject to secondary mutations that can restore their growth by making them more resistant to the drug. The *mar* locus that we have described does just that. The small increase in MIC to the fluoroquinolones is accompanied by a dramatic change in the MBC (Goldman et al 1996). With the *mar* locus active, more cells survive.

Spratt: This is actually what fluctuating levels should give you: the ability to just survive and not die. For instance, although group A streptococci have no mechanisms of resistance to penicillin, they have managed to develop tolerance, so they will survive. Then when the concentration goes down, off they go again.

Baquero: It is difficult to understand why *Streptococcus pyogenes* has not acquired penicillin resistance. However, a couple of years ago I came across an abstract from an Argentinean group showing that a penicillin binding protein modification in *S. pyogenes* led to a decrease in the bactericidal activity of penicillin. Our own group has observed in blood isolates a certain increase in the MIC to cephalothin during the last few years (Baquero 1994). I wonder whether these observations might represent the first step in the development of penicillin resistance.

Witte: It would be interesting to perform that sort of mixed culture experiment with TEM mutants in an *in vitro* model, to look at the pharmacokinetics over several generations. Has that been done?

Baquero: No, but that's a good suggestion.

Cohen: We talked yesterday about the increasing tendency for the use of drugs with infrequent dosing intervals. In a sense, some of the selective pressures of the extended-spectrum cephalosporins may be due to the fact that they are given infrequently and there is a much longer interval when drug levels are below those necessary for inhibition. What do we know about time intervals required for actual killing to occur? This seems to be a factor crucial to your 'ball' analogy (Fig. 1). If killing occurs in a few seconds to a few minutes, then a cidal level of an antibiotic achieved at a site will be sufficient to empty your container. If you are instead dealing with a small hole where they go out very slowly and your dosages are such that you don't really ever empty the container, the problem is made a lot worse. How long does it take to kill a bacterium?

Baquero: The differences in the selective activity of different antibiotics raises the concept of a 'selective window'. Certain concentrations are selective and not others.

Antibiotics, such as ceftriaxone, which maintain drug levels for much longer at lower concentrations than cefotaxime, may be more selective according to this model. On the other hand, pharmacokinetics may completely modify the system.

The killing time depends largely on the type of bacterium. For Gram-negatives, it takes a relatively long time and in fact depends on the time above the MIC. The average Gram-negative is killed in about an hour, in the case of cefotaxime.

Hall: It also depends on the antibiotic.

Spratt: For example, ampicillin lyses Gram-negative bacteria so they are dead within 20 min. Most of the newer β-lactams inhibit cell division, so killing may take a couple of hours. However, this is all in the lab, and the rate of killing in the human body is rather different.

Giamarellou: The problem with aminoglycosides is that we're trying to push the whole dose to once daily. How do you feel about the post-antibiotic effect? How would you correlate this with your experiments?

Baquero: Amikacin delivered with very high dosing intervals will be eventually selective or non-selective depending on the different mechanisms of resistance present in the bacteria involved in the infective process. In general, the aminoglycoside-modifying enzymes have a potent activity. It is rare to find low level antibiotic resistance to them, except if you are treating with a drug which is not very well inactivated. For instance, amikacin may select at low antibiotic concentrations strains harbouring Tn5, whose aminoglycoside phosphatidyltransferase determinants provide low-level resistance to this drug. The post-antibiotic effect is probably positive in terms of decreasing the selective power.

Giamarellou: According to your *in vitro* data, perhaps pharmaceutical companies should try to create liposomal compounds that deliver antibiotics in the compartments slowly but constantly. Alternatively, maybe we should try to find local delivery systems.

Baquero: The efficacy of local delivery systems to prevent the selection of resistance depends on the amount of drug released to the surroundings. For example, if you have sponges containing high antibiotic concentrations used to prevent wound infection, the concentrations are probably sufficient to prevent the survival of mutants. In general, the maintenance of high level antibiotic concentrations that are sufficient to suppress the growth of potentially emerging low-level resistant populations seems to be a good strategy.

Davies: I have a basic problem with many of the modelling studies; bacteria do not grow on Petri dishes in human beings. Many experiments done to determine MICs and MBCs of bacterial pathogens are misleading, because they have no relevance to actual drug treatment *in situ*.

I'd like to ask you about environmental aspects of antibiotic action. Aminoglycoside action is very sensitive to the concentration of sodium chloride. If there are variations in sodium chloride concentrations inside the body, what happens to MBCs and MICs?

Baquero: The local environment crucially affects the activity of the antibiotic. The redox potential, osmolarity or pH may modulate not only the activity of the antibiotic, but also the interaction between the antibiotic and the resistance enzyme (Culebras et al 1996). However, to understand this we need to have a much better idea of the microecological environment where antibiotics work.

Lenski: With regard to Julian Davies' comment about the problem with *in vitro* models, it seems to me that Fernando Baquero has shown very beautifully the power of the experimental system: it would be virtually impossible to have done something of this elegance *in vivo*. The general principle that his work demonstrates is extremely important and there's no reason to think it would not also apply *in vivo*. I also wanted to make something explicit that I think was implicit in his talk: the mathematics of the effect. If a population of 10^9 organisms is waiting for a double mutation that will give a high level resistance, you can calculate that it's going to take a very, very long time to get that rare double mutation event within a single cell, whether *in vivo* or *in vitro*. But if there is a selective advantage to cells having either single mutation alone, then a large population of intermediates can build up in a matter of days or weeks, which can then get the second mutation quite readily. The same point was brought out in the directed mutation debate, where some people were seeing double mutations and trying to understand how these could possibly be arising at such high frequency (Lenski & Mittler 1993). It turned out that there was subtle selection for an intermediate genotype with one mutation that allowed the accumulation of cells that could then quickly get the second mutation (Mittler & Lenski 1992). Ultimately, we want to understand natural systems, but as a test of theory showing how one can get a complicated adaptation — not fully formed but sequentially in steps — the work by Baquero is vital.

Bush: I've been intrigued for a long time by Dr Baquero's observations with these kinds of enzymes, especially with his TEM studies. One of the factors that we need to consider is that the most catalytically efficient TEM enzyme is the TEM-1 β-lactamase. Dr Baquero, have you looked for outer membrane changes in the strains that have been selected for, as to whether you may have a slight advantage that would then allow the TEM-1 to take over because it's a better enzyme than TEM-12?

Baquero: Remember that the selective effect was found after only 4 h of contact, and with the pre-prepared mutants. At the end of the experiment they had exactly the same outer membrane composition.

Cohen: It is rather ironic that with respect to antimicrobial design, two things that we have striven for — long half-life and broad spectrum — are probably two of the worst things with respect to the development of resistance.

Does this type of concentration effect come into play when you're talking about inducible resistance?

Baquero: Yes. I also did this sort of experiment with *Enterobacter cloacae* in the presence of different antibiotic concentrations. I did this with a wild-type strain that was mixed with a small proportion of a de-repressed variant constitutively producing chromosomal β-lactamase. This is obviously not inducible, but I expected the inducible forms to appear during the experiment. What happened is that essentially the advantage was for the de-repressed mutant. The inducible mutant tends to increase its proportion at certain concentrations, but was outnumbered by the induced cells at each selective concentration, even at low antibiotic concentrations, well below the MIC.

Lerner: Yesterday we talked about the pollution of the microbial environment from antibiotics in animal feed. Although that prophylactic practice may produce some benefit to balance the detrimental effects, it was difficult to evaluate the benefits in a clear manner. And difficult also to quantitate the deleterious effects on susceptibility among microbes. The prophylactic oral administration of a quinolone to patients undergoing bone marrow transplantation clearly produces a measurable benefit in markedly reducing the incidence of serious Gram-negative bacillary infections in these patients. Can we measure the cost of this pollution of the environment with quinolones?

Baquero: With quinolones we are paying an extremely high price at any level and not just in the body, but also in the inert environment. Quinolones are very stable, so when the patient goes to the toilet they excrete many of them which remain active in the sewage system. Our model of mixing up susceptible and resistant populations is probably a very sensitive system for detecting low antibiotic concentrations with potential selective effects in diluted environments. Low antibiotic concentrations could be sufficient to alter the quantitative composition of a mixture of susceptible and resistant organisms.

Levy: There are old studies with sewage systems which showed that during the settling period of the sewage the frequency of resistant bacteria increased (Grabow et al 1976). Some environmentalists call such systems breeding grounds for resistant bacteria.

Lerner: We ought to compare the sewage effluent from the cancer wards with that from the rest of the hospital with respect to the presence of quinolone resistance among aerobic Gram-negative bacilli.

References

Baquero F 1994 Antibiotic resistance in *Streptococcus pyogenes*. In: Pechère JC (ed) Acute bacterial pharyngitis. Cambridge Medical, Cambridge, p 81–87

Corpet DE, Lumeau S, Corpet F 1989 Minimum antibiotic levels for selecting a resistance plasmid in a gnotobiotic animal model. Antimicrob Agents Chemother 33:535–540

Culebras E, Martínez JL, Baquero F, Pérez-Díaz JC 1996 pH modulation of aminoglycoside resistance in *Staphylococcus epidermidis* harbouring 6′-N-aminoglycoside acetyltransferase. J Antimicrob Chemother 37:881–889

Gaynes R, Monnet D 1997 The contribution of antibiotic use on the frequency of antibiotic resistance in hospitals. In: Antibiotic resistance: origins, evolution, selection and spread. Wiley, Chichester (Ciba Found Symp 207) p 47–60

Goldman JD, White DG, Levy SB 1996 The multiple antibiotic resistance (*mar*) locus protects *Escherichia coli* from rapid cell killing by fluoroquinolones. Antimicrob Agents Chemother 40:1266–1269

Grabow WOK, van Zyk M, Prozesky OW 1976 Behavior in coventional sewage purification processes of coliform bacteria with transferable or non-transferable drug resistance. Water Res 10:717–723

Lenski RE, Mittler JE 1993 The directed mutation controversy and neo-Darwinism. Science 259:188–194

Mittler JE, Lenski RE 1992 Experimental evidence for an alternative to directed mutation in the *bgl* operon. Nature 356:446–448

Weinstein RA, Nathan C, Gruensfelde R, Kabins SA 1980 Endemic aminoglycoside resistance in gram-negative bacilli: epidemiology and mechanisms. J Infect Dis 141:338–341

The within-host population dynamics of antibacterial chemotherapy: conditions for the evolution of resistance

Marc Lipsitch and Bruce R. Levin

Department of Biology, Emory University, 1510 Clifton Road, Atlanta, GA 30322, USA

Abstract. For tuberculosis and a number of other bacterial infections, treatment with a single antimicrobial drug frequently fails due to the ascent of mutants resistant to that drug. To minimize the likelihood of this occurrence, multiple drugs with independent resistance mechanisms are used simultaneously. None the less, multiply resistant bacteria sometimes emerge even when patients are simultaneously treated with two or more drugs, and the ascent of these multiply-resistant mutants may result in treatment failure in the patient and spread of these resistant bacteria to other hosts. We consider two mathematical models of antibacterial chemotherapy which can account for the ascent of multiple antibiotic resistance within hosts treated with multiple antibiotics. In both, multiple resistance evolves because of selection favouring mutants resistant to fewer than all of the chemotherapeutic agents employed, *intermediates*. In one model, this occurs because of temporal fluctuations in the concentrations of the antibiotics in the course of normal treatment and/or because of non-adherence to the treatment regime. In the other, intermediates are favoured and multiple resistance evolves because of tissue and somatic cell heterogeneity in the effective concentrations of the antibiotics and physiological variation in the sensitivity of subpopulations of bacteria to different antibiotics. We discuss the limitations (and assets) of this model and approach and the implications for the design of antibiotic treatment regimes. Finally, we consider how the assumptions behind this model and the predictions made from its analysis could be tested experimentally.

1997 Antibiotic resistance: origins, evolution, selection and spread. Wiley, Chichester (Ciba Foundation Symposium 207) p 112–130

In contrast to the extensive and growing literature on the molecular and genetic mechanisms of bacterial resistance to antibiotics, relatively little is known about the population biological processes underlying the emergence of antibiotic resistance. For several important infections (notably those with *Mycobacterium* and *Pseudomonas*) single-drug treatment often fails as the result of the outgrowth of resistant strains. A general strategy to deal with this resistance problem is to treat simultaneously with multiple antibiotics for which bacteria do not show cross-resistance. The idea behind these multidrug treatment protocols is appealing. While bacterial lineages resistant to single drugs may be present as rare variants at the start of treatment, or emerge soon after, the frequency of bacteria simultaneously resistant to more than one of these agents would be negligible, on the order of the product of the frequencies of the lineages resistant to single drugs. Nevertheless, multidrug antibacterial chemotherapy may also fail because of the ascent of bacteria resistant to some or all of the antibiotics used for treatment. This situation is particularly problematic in tuberculosis chemotherapy (Mitchison 1984, 1992) but has been observed with multidrug treatment of other bacterial infections (Fish et al 1995).

One possible explanation for the failure of multidrug antibacterial chemotherapy is that the assumptions behind these treatment protocols are not met in treated patients. Implicit in the logic behind multidrug therapy is the assumption that in the presence of all the different antibiotics, lineages resistant to fewer than all the drugs employed would not be able to proliferate. If populations of these '*intermediates*' were able to proliferate during the course of treatment, their numbers could eventually become sufficient for mutants resistant to additional drugs to be produced, thereby setting the stage for the clinical emergence of multiple drug resistance.

In this report, we review the results of experiments of antibiotic inhibition of bacterial growth and recent mathematical models designed to examine the effects of temporal and spatial variation in antibiotic efficacy on the selection of intermediates during multiple drug therapy.[1] We explore the a priori conditions under which these sources of variation will favour bacteria resistant to some, but not all of the drugs employed for treatment and the contribution of non-adherence (non-compliance) to treatment failure due to the evolution of multiple resistance. We discuss the empirical fit of these models and the implications of these theoretical results for the development of antibiotic treatment protocols. Finally, and most importantly, we describe how the validity of the assumptions behind these models and their predictions can be tested experimentally.

Temporal variation in antibiotic concentration

In vitro observations

Traditionally, the effectiveness of an antimicrobial agent against a particular strain of bacteria is characterized by a single summary parameter, the minimal inhibitory concentration (MIC). This is the lowest concentration that prevents visible growth of an inoculum incubated for 16–20 h under defined conditions (Pratt & Fekety 1986). The use of this single parameter obscures the fact that in almost all cases the inhibitory or killing effect of a particular antibiotic is a continuously varying function of its concentration. E. R. Garrett and collaborators have measured the

---

[1]To a large extent, but not entirely, the substance of this report is a review of material presented in two, at the time of this writing submitted, articles (Lipsitch & Levin 1997a,b). Further details of these models and the analysis of their properties can be found in those reports.

relationship between drug concentration and apparent growth rate (the difference between the cell division rate and rate of cell death, either or both of which may themselves be functions of antibiotic concentration) for a number of antibiotics (Garrett 1971, 1978, Garrett & Miller 1965, Garrett & Won 1973, Garrett & Wright 1967). This relationship may take a number of forms, for example, linear or saturating, but in each case there is a region in which net rate of growth declines continuously. For bacteriostatic antibiotics, the net growth rate reaches a minimum at zero; for bactericidal drugs, it becomes negative at sufficiently high concentration. Depending on the drug, there may also be ranges of very low or very high concentrations in which increases in dose have no effect on the apparent growth rate. At the low end, this may be due to binding of low concentrations of antibiotic and at the high end it may be attributable to saturation of antibiotic receptors. The breadth of the range of concentrations for which increases in concentration increase the effectiveness of the antibiotic may vary widely between classes of antibiotics (Vogelman et al 1988) but such a range seems to exist in virtually all cases. The concentration-dependent effects of antibiotics have important consequences for the population dynamics of susceptible and resistant bacteria *in vivo*. Concentrations of antibiotics decline between doses and in many cases fall below the MIC for some portion of the dosing interval, allowing some regrowth of bacterial populations. The changes in populations reflect the net effects of antibiotic-mediated killing over a range of concentrations and any regrowth that occurs at low concentrations.

To illustrate this phenomenon, we present the results of some of our own experiments on the growth of an *E. coli* 018:K1:H7 (CAB1, obtained from C. Bloch) in Luria broth with streptomycin. After allowing 1 ml of overnight culture to grow for 30 min in 10 ml of antibiotic-free broth, an aliquot was added at a ratio of 1:50 to broth containing different concentrations of streptomycin. Samples were taken at periodic intervals and the optical density (600 nm) of the culture and the viable cell density estimated respectively with a spectrophotometer and by serial dilution and plating on LB (Luria Bertoni) agar to determine the number of colony forming units (CFUs).

The results of these experiments are presented in Fig. 1. The rate of cell division, as estimated by optical density, declines with increasing concentrations of streptomycin (Fig. 1a). While there is the suggestion of a limited amount of growth with 23.3 µg/ml streptomycin, above 26.7 µg/ml there is no apparent increase in the density of the culture after the second sample. The colony count data not only confirm this, but also indicate that above 20 µg/ml streptomycin causes a net decline in the bacterial population, and the rate and extent of this mortality increases with increasing concentration (Fig. 1b). On the other hand, this bactericidal effect of streptomycin is short-lived. After a period of time the colony count density levels-off and eventually, the population of bacteria recovers. By 24 h, there is essentially no difference in the live cell density of the cultures containing streptomycin and their antibiotic-free controls. Additional experiments, performed in collaboration with Tomoko Steen, Nina Walker and Fred Rege, suggest that this levelling-off and reversal in the bactericidal activity of streptomycin is a consequence of decay in the effective concentration of streptomycin in Luria broth maintained at 37 °C.

(a)

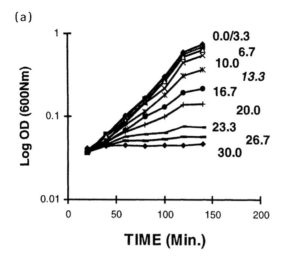

(b)

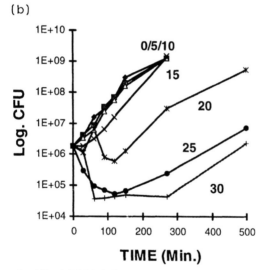

FIG. 1.   Growth of *E. coli* CAB1 (018:K1:H7) in Luria broth with streptomycin. (a) Changes in optical density (600 nm) with different concentrations (μg/ml) of streptomycin. (b) Changes in the number of colony forming units (CFUs) with different concentrations of streptomycin.

A model of treatment with temporal variation in antibiotic concentration

In Fig. 2, we present a diagram of the basic model of antibiotic treatment employed in Lipsitch & Levin (1997a). The host is infected with bacteria that are, respectively, sensitive and resistant to a single antibiotic, with densities, S and $R1$, bacteria per ml.

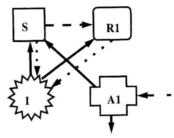

FIG. 2.   Model of immune and antibiotic control of a growing population of bacteria. *S*, density of antibiotic sensitive bacteria; *R*, density of antibiotic resistant bacteria; *I*, intensity of the immune response; *A*, concentration of the antibiotic. The bacterial populations replicate and stimulate the immune response at a rate proportional to the total density. This specific immune response, in turn, kills both antibiotic sensitive and resistant bacteria at a rate directly proportional to its intensity (level) *I*. The antibiotic inhibits the growth of and kills only sensitive bacteria.

In the absence of a specific immune response, both populations grow at constant rates, r and r′, which reflect the action of the non-specific defences like cytotoxic compounds in serum on the rate of growth of the bacteria. The population of bacteria stimulates the facultative, specific immune defences to increase in intensity, *I*, at a rate that is a function of the density of the total population of bacteria. Antibiotic sensitive and resistant bacteria are equally subject to killing by the specific immune defence, which occurs at a rate proportional to *I*. The antibiotic is present at a concentration *A 1* and is metabolized or removed from the host at a constant rate *k*, which is independent of the density of bacteria. The antibiotic kills sensitive bacteria at a rate proportional to its concentration but has no effect on the growth of the resistant population. Periodically, a fixed dose of antibiotic is administered to the host.

The basic model can be extended to account for treatment with any number of antibiotics. Bacteria may be sensitive or resistant to each antibiotic administered, so that with *n* different antibiotics there are 2^n possible populations with different resistance profiles. The interactions among multiple antibiotics in their effects on the net growth of bacteria may be complex in reality. In this paper, we describe the results that stem from the assumption that drugs act additively; in a more detailed paper (Lipsitch & Levin 1997a), we describe the effects of other assumptions.

Results

In our analysis of the properties of this model, we consider three different kinds of infections:

(A) Self-limiting. The rate at which the specific immune system response increases in magnitude and its maximum intensity, I_{max}, are sufficient to clear the infection without antibiotics.

(B) Level compromised. At its maximum intensity, I_{max}, the immune response is not sufficient to clear the infection.

(C) Rate compromised. The maximum intensity of the immune response, I_{max}, is sufficient to clear the infection in the absence of treatment, but the intensity of the immune response grows too slowly for the bacterial population to be cleared before it reaches a lethal density.

In the following paragraphs, we summarize our primary conclusions (predictions) for situations where there is full compliance with the treatment regime (Lipsitch & Levin 1996a).

Resistance and treatment failure with single drug therapy. If a single drug is employed and mutants resistant to it are not already present when treatment is initiated, they are unlikely to arise during treatment as long as the combined effects of the antibiotic and the host response produce a net decline in the sensitive bacterial population at a rate comparable to the rate of cell division.

If resistant mutants are already present or arise during treatment, they will increase in frequency in the bacterial population. In the case of a self-limiting, type A infection, as long as resistant bacteria are a small minority, treatment will reduce the peak density of the bacterial population and may thereby reduce morbidity of the infection. For infections where the peak immune response is too low to control the infection, type B, if resistant mutants are present at all, they will ascend, resulting in treatment failure. In a rate-compromised, type C infection, the qualitative outcome of treatment depends on the initial sizes and rate of growth of the sensitive and resistant bacterial populations, the rate of mutation to resistance, the rate at which the specific immune system responds the growing population of bacteria, the efficacy (inhibitory/killing effect) of the antibiotics, and the maximum density of bacteria that can be tolerated by the host. In some cases, even with substantial numbers of resistant bacteria, in an infection in a rate-compromised host that would otherwise achieve lethal densities, antibiotic treatment will buy sufficient time to allow the immune system to clear the infection.

Resistance and treatment failure with multi-drug therapy. We restricted our formal consideration of multiple drug therapy to type B infections and two drugs. While single drug treatment of this type of infection will fail if mutants resistant to that drug are present, therapy with two drugs can prevent this outcome, even if mutants resistant to each single drug are present at substantial frequencies. For successful treatment under these conditions, it is essential that bacteria simultaneously resistant to both drugs do not arise. To prevent them from being generated, it is necessary to treat in such a way that each antibiotic causes a net decline in the density of the bacterial population resistant to the other drug. If this is accomplished, then the chances of generating a doubly-resistant mutant are low, just as the chances of generating a singly-resistant mutant would be low if a fully sensitive population were to be treated successfully. In cases where intermediates can ascend, the model predicts that the first resistant lineages to ascend will be those resistant to the most effective antibiotic, i.e. the one which alone would cause the greatest net decline in the density of bacteria sensitive to it. This prediction may be modified if the replication rates of resistant bacteria differ greatly from those of sensitive bacteria.

Non-adherence. We considered two ways by which a patient may deviate from a prescribed treatment regime. The first we call 'random non-adherence': the patient occasionally neglects to take the drugs at the prescribed time. For convenience we assume that the probability P that drugs will not be taken at a particular time $(0 < P \leqslant 1)$ is constant and that treatment is missed completely. The patient does not compensate for this omission by taking greater doses of the drug at the next dosing interval or by taking the drug(s) at times other than the scheduled treatment interval. In the second non-adherence scheme we considered, 'thermostat non-adherence,' the patient stops taking the drug when the total bacterial population falls below some lower threshold and resumes when the population reaches an upper threshold. The idea behind this non-adherence scheme is that the symptoms of the infection are directly correlated with the density of bacteria. When that density falls below a particular level, the patient no longer has the symptoms which motivated treatment, and the side-effects or other considerations dissuade the patient from taking these drugs in the absence of symptoms. Our consideration of non-adherence was restricted solely to type B infections, where treatment is essential to clear the infection and the bacterial population will grow unchecked if multiply-resistant mutants arise.

In both cases, by promoting the growth and/or maintenance of intermediates resistant to fewer than all the drugs employed, non-adherence can result in treatment failure due to multiple resistance in an otherwise effective multi-antibiotic treatment regime. The manner in which this occurs differs for the random and thermostat models of non-adherence. For the random model, the effect of non-adherence is analogous to that of taking the same dose regularly but at a reduced frequency. The presence of antibiotics provides selection pressure favouring the preferential survival and growth of resistant mutants, while the reduced frequency permits longer periods of regrowth of the bacterial population between doses. If non-adherence is frequent enough, this may permit a net increase in the numbers of intermediates during treatment.

With the thermostat model, the absolute densities of these intermediates may decline while the drugs are being taken, but because of the advantage intermediates have in the presence of antibiotics, the relative frequencies of these resistant bacteria will increase during each treatment period. During each successive period of non-adherence, the bacterial population will re-grow, maintaining the increased proportion of resistant mutants (though this may decline somewhat during non-adherence if resistant mutants grow more slowly than their susceptible counterparts). With enough cycles of drug-taking and non-adherence, the densities of these singly-resistant mutants will eventually be sufficiently large for mutants resistant to the second antibiotic to arise in their population, thus generating the first doubly-resistant lineages.

This process of enrichment depends on an increase in the proportion of singly-resistant bacteria during each period of adherence. If the population of singly-resistant bacteria goes extinct during each period of drug-taking, then the enrichment will not occur. A key parameter regulating the likelihood of such extinctions is the net difference in fitness between sensitive and singly-resistant bacteria. This quantity is greatest when resistant bacteria grow (in the absence of drugs) at the same rate as susceptible ones, and when drug activities are additive or super-additive, so that susceptible bacteria are killed more rapidly than singly resistant ones in the presence of drugs. Less-than-additive drug action, or high fitness costs of resistance, will retard or may even prevent the enrichment process.

Spatial heterogeneity in antibiotic action

It is reasonable to anticipate that at any time, the concentrations of antibiotics will vary among the different tissues of a treated host, and the effectiveness of a particular antibiotic may depend on the tissue and/or somatic cells in which the bacteria are located as well as the bacteria's own physiological state. For bacterial infections that are widely disseminated within a particular tissue or set of tissues in a host, such as infections with *Mycobacterium tuberculosis*, such heterogeneity may play an especially important role in antibiotic treatment.

Mitchison (1979, 1984) has proposed that the mycobacteria within a particular host can be subdivided into a number of distinct, though fluid, subpopulations, each of which responds to various antibiotics in different ways. Mitchison's scheme is depicted in Fig. 3. In this model, there is one, large mycobacterial population that is growing rapidly and is susceptible to isoniazid, rifampin, streptomycin and other drugs commonly used to treat tuberculosis. A second population alternates between a resting phase and 'spurts of metabolism' and is physiologically insensitive to all of these drugs except rifampin; a third, acid-inhibited population is affected almost exclusively by pyrazinamide. These phenotypic/physiological forms of drug-insensitivity are distinct from the kind of genetically determined resistance we have been discussing. As Mitchison & Nunn (1986) have observed, however, phenotypic insulation from drug action may contribute to the development of genetically determined resistance. The 'protected populations' sensitive only to one drug are, in effect, experiencing single-drug therapy, with a corresponding risk of selecting for genetic resistance to that drug. For example, a mutant resistant to rifampin would be able to survive and perhaps even multiply (albeit slowly) in 'spurts of metabolism' unchecked by any drug. However, such mutants would be killed if they began growing rapidly, since isoniazid would then become effective against them.

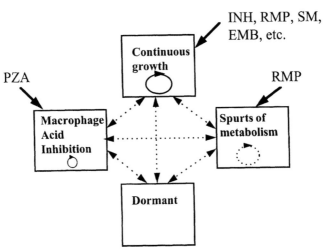

FIG. 3.   A model of multiple antibiotic treatment of tuberculosis. EMB, ethambutol; INH, isoniazid; PZA, pyrazinamide; RMP, rifampin; SM, streptomycin. Solid lines indicate the loss (killing) of bacteria and the broken lines migration between different subhabitats. This figure is adapted from the model of tuberculosis chemotherapy proposed by Mitchison (1979).

A model of spatial heterogeneity in antibiotic action

To illustrate how and in what circumstances spatial heterogeneity in antibiotic efficacy may favour the evolution of intermediates and to better understand the quantitative conditions under which this will occur, we developed a simple mathematical model of this process. In this model, there are two compartments, A and B, which contain N_A and N_B bacteria growing at rates r_A and r_B, respectively. Bacteria from the A compartment migrate to B at rate m_A and migrate from B to A at rate m_B (Fig. 4). Migration in this context is not limited to physical translocation within an infected lung, but refers to any change of physiological, metabolic, or environmental state that results in a change in drug susceptibility. In this model, unlike the previous one, we assume that at least when treatment is initiated, the host immune responses are operating at a constant level. The killing of bacteria by these specific and general host defences and antibiotics are reflected in the magnitudes of the growth rates, r_A and r_B.

Results

In this linear model, each population of bacteria with a particular resistance profile (for example, bacteria sensitive to all antibiotics, or bacteria resistant to antibiotic 1 and sensitive to antibiotic 2, and so on) can be considered separately. Obviously, in such a system, if a population of bacteria can grow in both compartments, then it will grow in the system as a whole; if it experiences net killing in both compartments, its

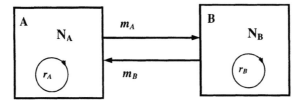

FIG. 4.   Two-compartment model of antibiotic treatment. Bacteria, of densities N_A and N_B replicate at rates, r_A and r_B in two separate habitats, A and B. Bacteria from the B habitat migrate to A at a rate m_A and those from B, migrate to A at a rate m_B. For our analysis of the properties of this model, we assume that two antibiotics are used for treatment, both of which kill bacteria in compartment A, the 'unprotected' compartment. Only one of these antibiotics kills bacteria in compartment B, the 'protected' compartment.

population as a whole will decline. In the case where a population of bacteria is able to grow in one 'protected' compartment (say, compartment B) but is killed in the other, 'unprotected' compartment (say, compartment A), the condition for the population as a whole to experience net growth is:

$$r_B > \frac{r_A m_B}{r_A - m_A} \qquad (1)$$

One important feature of this condition is that net growth will always occur if the growth rate in the protected compartment is greater than the migration rate out of it. Therefore, if migration out of the compartment is slow, then net growth may occur, even if killing is very efficient in the unprotected compartment and growth is slow in the protected compartment.

The model can be used to consider a simplified version of the situation envisaged by Mitchison (1979). Restricting our attention for the present to just the main, growing population and the population showing 'spurts' of metabolism, it is clear that 'wild-type' bacteria, bearing no resistance genes, will decline in both populations, since they will be affected by rifampin everywhere and by other drugs if they are in the growing phase. The same is true of many of the other 'intermediates' that may be present in the population — for example, isoniazid-resistant or streptomycin-resistant bacteria. Rifampin-resistant bacteria, however, will be able to grow if they do so by 'spurts of metabolism,' although they will be killed if they enter the rapidly dividing population. Such growth will be considerably slower than active growth (Dickinson & Mitchison 1981) and may, in fact, be almost negligible (D. A. Mitchison, personal communication 1996). If bacteria do grow in the protected compartment, albeit at a very low rate, condition (1) determines whether rifampin-resistant bacteria will ascend and eventually give rise to a doubly resistant mutant. For example, let us assume B is the 'protected' compartment where only rifampin is active, while A is the main population, where active replication makes the bacteria susceptible to both drugs. We further assume the migration rates of $m_A = m_B = 0.005$ per hour and that the net rate at which rifampin-resistant mutants are killed by isoniazid is $r_A = -0.07$ per hour (Jindani et al 1980). Then from (1) we can see that the overall population of rifampin-resistant mutants will grow as long as their growth rate in the protected compartment, r_B, exceeds a rate of 0.0047 per hour.

Finite compartment size.   The model above is more realistic if one adds the assumption that the protected compartment may be of limited size. This can be accomplished by adding a 'carrying capacity' to compartment B — limiting the rate of proliferation of bacteria in the compartment and the rate of migration into the compartment when the total population approaches the carrying capacity. We performed simulations in a model with such an assumption, using parameters that satisfied condition (1), so that with an unlimited protected compartment[2], resistance would emerge. We ran a series of simulations carrying capacities for compartment B of 10^4 and 10^8. These simulations were initiated solely with sensitive bacteria and, in the absence of resistant mutants, terminate with the infection being cleared. With a carrying capacity in compartment B of 10^4, no resistant mutants arose in 100 simulations. With those same parameters and a carrying capacity of 10^8, single and then double resistant mutants arose in 16 out of the 100 runs. This confirms the intuition that limiting the size of the protected compartment lowers the likelihood of the emergence of resistance. In the 16 runs where treatment failed, resistance first arose to the antibiotic that was effective in both compartments, drug 2, and on average the doubly resistant mutants first appeared 5570 h after the start of treatment.

The effects of non-adherence.   In our analysis of the properties of this model we also considered the 'thermostat' scheme of non-adherence, where the patient stops taking drugs when the total density of the bacterial population falls below some pre-

---

[2]Parameters:
Drug 1 (isoniazid) is active in compartment A only; Drug 2 (rifampin) is active in both compartment A and compartment B.
Sensitive strain:
$b_B=0.1$, $b_B=0.01$, $d_A=0.35$, $d_B=0.022$, $r_A=-0.25$, $r_B=-0.012$.
Strain resistant to drug 1:
$b_A=0.09$, $b_B0.009$, $d_A=0.15$, $d_B=0.02$, $r_A=-0.06$, $r_B=-0.011$.
Strain resistant to drug 2:
$b_A=0.09$, $b_B=0.009$, $d_A=0.2$, $d_B=0.002$, $r_A=-0.11$, $r_B=0.007$.
Strain resistant to both drugs
$b_A=0.081$, $b_B=0.0081$, $d_A=0$, $d_B=0$.
Mutation rates for resistance to drug 1: 3×10^{-7}.
Mutation rates for resistance to drug 2: 2.5×10^{-9}.
All strains: $m_A=m_B=0.002$. In these simulations, the population in the host at large is allowed to grow untreated ($d = 0$ for all strains in both compartments) until they reach 10^9, at which point treatment begins.

determined level and doesn't start treatment again until that density reaches an also specified higher level, respectively 10^4 and 10^9 in our simulations.

The parameter values used for these non-adherence simulations are the same as those described above and in footnote 2. With non-adherence and a protected compartment carrying capacity of either 10^4 or 10^8, resistant mutants arose and treatment failed in all 100 simulations. The dynamics and time of ascent of the single and double resistant mutants in these non-adherence simulations varied with the carrying capacity of the protected compartment. In all 100 runs with a carrying capacity of 10^4, the first mutants to reach high levels were resistant to drug 1 (active only in the unprotected compartment), and the first doubly-resistant mutant arose on average at 592 time units. With non-adherence and a compartment B carrying capacity of 10^8, resistance to the sole antibiotic effective in the protected compartment, drug 2, arose first and on average it took 4400 h before the doubly-resistant mutants first appeared. Interestingly, with the larger protected compartment, the order of ascent of resistance changed, and the rate of ascent was much slower than with the small protected compartment. This is because the ascent of mutants resistant to the drug effective in the protected compartment is very slow, corresponding to the very slow growth achievable in this protected compartment.

The effect of mutation rate. On first consideration it may seem that with multiple antibiotic therapy, the order at which resistance arises would depend on rates at which bacteria generate resistance to the different antibiotics. As can be seen above, that is not necessarily the case. In the above simulation, resistance to the drug 1 occurred at a rate of 2.5×10^{-7} while resistance to the drug 2 occurred at a rate of 3×10^{-9}. Nevertheless, in several simulations, resistance to drug 2 arose first. Furthermore, when the simulations described were repeated with the rates of mutation switched (so that the antibiotic active in both compartments had a mutation rate of 2.5×10^{-7} and the antibiotic active only in the unprotected compartment had a mutation rate of 3×10^{-9}), the results were similar to those with the original mutation rates in most cases, suggesting that, for these parameters, at least, differences in selection are more important than even a rather large differential in mutation rates. (The results of these simulations are reported fully in Lipsitch & Levin [1997b].)

Discussion

Combined pharmacokinetic/pharmacodynamic modelling has been advanced as a technique for predicting the *in vivo* effects of various dosing regimens on a population of bacteria susceptible to a particular antimicrobial drug. These techniques have had some success despite the complexities of drug–host interactions, post-antibiotic effects, and other complications. However, such models have not been used to propose and test quantitative mechanisms for the emergence of resistance (Nolting & Derendorf 1995). These mathematical and simulation studies represent a first attempt at such quantitative understanding of how and when resistance will emerge. The common theme of these models is that multiple resistance emerges because singly-resistant mutants, present at or near the start of treatment, are able to grow even though the majority population is controlled by an antibiotic or combination of antibiotics. This may occur as a result of temporal heterogeneity in drug concentrations that results from fluctuating drug concentrations between doses and/or non-adherence to the treatment regime. It may also occur as a result of spatial heterogeneity in drug penetration or efficacy. Any of these mechanisms alone may be sufficient to cause the failure of a treatment regime that would otherwise succeed, and they may work synergistically to cause or speed the ascent of multiple resistance.

The direct consequence of these hypotheses is that preventing the emergence of resistance depends on the suppression, not only of the majority population, which will be (in ideal circumstances) susceptible to all of the drugs employed, but also to singly-resistant subpopulations, which are none the less (in the case of multidrug therapy) susceptible to one or more other drugs used. If these hypotheses are correct, then, to prevent the emergence of resistance, the effect of each drug alone, rather than their synergistic-additive effect will be the crucial parameter.

An important common prediction of these models is that the strength of selection for these 'intermediates' will be a dominant force in determining the rate and order of the ascent of resistance. This provides an alternative explanation for such phenomena as the change in resistance patterns in tuberculosis observed in HIV-infected patients, for which changes in mutation rates have already been advanced as one hypothesis (Nolan et al 1995, Bradford et al 1996).

Limitations and tests. These models are, obviously, only simple caricatures of bacterial infections, the immune response and the pharmacokinetics, physiology and population dynamics of antibiotic treatment. We could wax extensively, if not elegantly, about the limitations of these models, the way we analysed their properties and the values of the parameters employed. In Lipsitch & Levin (1997a,b) we have discussed these caveats at some length. We refer the reader to these more detailed and technical reports for these discussions of the limitations of these models and our analyses of their properties.

An important virtue of these models is that the validity of the assumptions behind their construction and the predictions derived from their analysis can be tested with experimental animals. The most critical of these predictions for the evolution of multiple resistance is that populations of mutants resistant to fewer than all the antibiotics employed for treatment — intermediates — can grow in hosts periodically treated with multiple antibiotics, even if these are administered in doses that are effective against the majority population of bacteria that is sensitive to both agents. One way to test this is to inoculate a number of mice, or other laboratory mammals, with mixtures containing high concentrations of antibiotic-sensitive bacteria and relatively low frequencies of mutants resistant to one or more antibiotic used for treatment. Treatment could be initiated immediately or at different times after the infecting bacteria become established, and bacteria sampled at the site of the infection as well as other tissues, such as the spleen, liver and blood. The densities of sensitive and resistant bacteria could be estimated by dilution and plating. Both temporal variation and spatial heterogeneity models predict that these intermediates will increase in relative frequency, and in some cases in absolute numbers, even under treatment that is effective against the majority, sensitive population.

The temporal heterogeneity model predicts that for effective combination therapy in the presence of singly-resistant mutants, the dose of each drug required to prevent the emergence of resistance will be greater than or equal to that which would be necessary for effective monotherapy in the absence of resistant mutants. This prediction may well be incorrect, particularly if the ability of the immune system to clear small numbers of (resistant) bacteria is greater than its ability to clear large numbers of bacteria. Testing this prediction and elucidating the reasons for its failure, if it proves incorrect, will provide important insights into the population dynamics underlying the emergence of resistance.

Implications for treatment and the epidemiology of resistance. In their present state, these models are simply elaborate hypotheses; it is necessary to test them in animals before assessing their implications for treatment and epidemiology. None the less, given the difficulty of measuring many of the important parameters of infections in human or animal hosts, and the need to rely on informed hypotheses in refining methods of treatment and interpreting data, it is worthwhile to consider some broad implications of models like the ones presented here. These interpretations, while tentative, may suggest further experimental work to test the interpretations.

The spatial heterogeneity model predicts that differences in antibiotic efficacy between compartments are most likely to lead to the rise of resistance when the 'protected' population is large and when it grows rapidly in comparison to the rate of 'migration' into unprotected populations and the rate of killing in the unprotected populations. In so far as protection from drug efficacy results from very slow or even zero growth (Mitchison 1979), 'effective monotherapy' of protected populations is unlikely to lead to the ascent of resistance. This may account for the fact that in tuberculosis, resistance rarely emerges to drugs active against such protected populations. Furthermore, when such resistance does emerge, it seems to occur under special circumstances that may lead to these favourable conditions: where protection occurs due to failure of drug penetration, which may permit effective monotherapy against rapidly growing mycobacterial populations (Elliott et al 1995), or in cases of immunocompromised hosts (Nolan et al 1995, Bradford et al 1996), in whom growth rates or population sizes may be greater.

The model of temporal heterogeneity suggests that it may be useful to think of infections where resistance may emerge as three concurrent infections (in the case of two-drug therapy) — a large-scale infection of sensitive bacteria, plus a much smaller infection with bacteria resistant to each of the two drugs individually. The model suggests the most conservative/pessimistic assumption about such infections — that treating each of these infections will not aid in clearing the others. As a result, therapy must be adequate to clear each population individually, or the risk of emergence of resistance remains. Further work testing this conservative assumption will likely reveal interesting mechanisms at work in real infections.

These modelling and experimental efforts address only one part of the growing antibiotic resistance problem — the selection of resistant, pathogenic organisms within an individual host — which may have consequences both for an individual patient and for the spread of resistant infections to other patients. The epidemiological importance of the spread of resistant microbes selected in a single treated patient has been clearly documented in tuberculosis (Bifani et al 1996) and may be important in other infections as well. By contrast, for colonizing or commensal organisms that cause disease in a minority of colonized hosts, the spread of resistance will be more closely related to the use of antibiotics to treat infections caused by other organisms.

Acknowledgements

We wish to thank T. Steen, N. Walker, R. Antia and F. Rege for sharing their data on the denaturation of streptomycin. We also want to express our gratitude to D. A. Mitchison for providing both the inspiration for some of this endeavour, and for his critical and very useful commentary about our interpretation of his model of tuberculosis chemotherapy. This endeavour has been supported by a research grant from the National Institutes of Health, GM33782.

References

Bifani PJ, Plikaytis BB, Kapur V et al 1996 Origin and interstate spread of a New York City multi-drug-resistant *Mycobacterium tuberculosis* clone family. JAMA 275:452–457

Bradford WZ, Martin JN, Reingold AL, Schecter GF, Hopewell PC, Small PM 1996 The changing epidemiology of acquired drug-resistant tuberculosis in San Francisco, USA. Lancet 348:928–931

Dickinson JM, Mitchison DA 1981 Experimental models to explain the high sterilizing activity of rifampin in the chemotherapy of tuberculosis. Am Rev Respir Dis 123:367–371

Elliott AM, Berning SE, Iseman MD, Peloquin CA 1995 Failure of drug penetration and acquisition of drug resistance in chronic tuberculous empyema. Tubercle Lung Dis 76:463–467

Fish DN, Piscitelli SC, Danziger LH 1995 Development of resistance during antimicrobial therapy: a review of antibiotic classes and patient characteristics in 173 studies. Pharmacotherapy 15:279–291

Garrett ER 1971 Drug action and assay by microbial kinetics. Prog Drug Res 15:271–352

Garrett ER 1978 Kinetics of antimicrobial action. Scand J Infect Dis (suppl) 14:54–85

Garrett ER, Miller GH 1965 Kinetics and mechanisms of action of antibiotics on microorganisms. III. The inhibitory action of tetracycline and chloramphenicol on *Escherichia coli* established by total and viable counts. J Pharmacol Sci 54:427

Garrett ER, Won CM 1973 Kinetics and mechanisms of drug action on microorganisms. XVII. Bactericidal effects of penicillin, kanamycin, and rifampin with and without organism pretreatment with bacteriostatic chloramphenicol, tetracycline and novobiocin. J Pharmacol Sci 62:1666–1673

Garrett ER, Wright OK 1967 Kinetics and mechanisms of action of drugs on microorganisms. VII. Quantitative adherence of sulfonamide action on microbial growth to a receptor-site model. J Pharmacol Sci 56:1576–1585

Jindani A, Aber VR, Edwards EA, Mitchison DA 1980 The early bactericidal activity of drugs in patients with pulmonary tuberculosis. Am Rev Respir Dis 121:939–949

Lipsitch M, Levin BR 1997a The population dynamics of antimicrobial chemotherapy. Antimicrob Agents Chemother 41:363–373

Lipsitch M, Levin BR 1997b The population dynamics of tuberculosis chemotherapy: on the role of bacterial population heterogeneity in the emergence of resistance. Submitted to Tubercle and Lung Dis

Mitchison DA 1979 Basic mechanisms of chemotherapy. Chest 76:771–781

Mitchison DA 1984 Drug resistance in mycobacteria. Br Med Bull 40:84–90

Mitchison DA 1992 The Garrod Lecture. Understanding the chemotherapy of tuberculosis — current problems. J Antimicrob Chemother 29:477–493

Mitchison DA, Nunn AJ 1986 Influence of initial drug resistance on the response to short-course chemotherapy of pulmonary tuberculosis. Am Rev Respir Dis 133:423–430

Nolan CM, Williams DL, Cave MD et al 1995 Evolution of rifampin resistance in human immunodeficiency virus–associated tuberculosis. Am J Respir Crit Care Med 152:1067–1071

Nolting A, Derendorf H 1995 Pharmacokinetic/pharmacodynamic modeling of antibiotics. In: Derendorf H, Hochhaus G (eds) Handbook of pharmacokinetic/pharmacodynamic correlation. CRC Press, Boca Raton, FL, p 363–388

Pratt WB, Fekety R 1986 The antimicrobial drugs. Oxford University Press, New York

Vogelman B, Gudmundsson S, Leggett J, Turnidge J, Ebert S, Craig WA 1988 Correlation of antimicrobial pharmacokinetic parameters with therapeutic efficacy in an animal model. J Infect Dis 158:831–847

DISCUSSION

Summers: What's your relative weighting for the contributions to killing of the immune system and the antibiotic you used?

Levin: In one form of the model, we assume the immune system at its maximum level is unable to control the infection and antibiotics are essential for clearance. In another form of the model (really the same model with different parameters) we assume that the outcome depends on the joint action of the immune system and the antibiotic and that at its maximum level, the immune system can control the infection by itself. Under these conditions, the antibiotic increases the rate of clearance but is not essential for that clearance.

Summers: But is your immune system at a constant threshold, above which you add the antibiotic effect?

Levin: No. In the model the intensity level of the immune response increases in time at a rate proportional to the density of the infecting population of bacteria, the antigen.

Summers: But, if you took labels off them, would a contribution from a unit of the immune system be equivalent to a contribution of a unit of antibiotic?

Levin: That depends on the concentration of the antibiotic and the intensity of the immune response at that time. For a while, the extent of antibiotic inhibition of bacterial growth can exceed that of the immune system. The relative contributions of these two factors in the control of the infection are continually changing. The inducible immune response function used in this model is the same as that Rustom Antia, Bob May and I published a few years ago (Antia et al 1994). We are just now beginning to examine its validity; it is already clear-cut from the experiments done by one of my graduate students, Terry de Rouin, who has injected *E. coli* K1 (018:K1:H7) into the thighs of mice, that the inducible form of host defence considered in this model is only part of the story. Terry's studies suggest that the non-specific phagocytic cells must also be considered. In these experiments, early in the infectious process the phagocytic cells probably play the dominant role in determining whether the mouse will live or not.

Baquero: To some extent, your model considers the immune system to be behaving similarly to an antibiotic. When the bacterial population is increasing, immunity is rising. That is like a higher dosage of antibiotic or a new antibiotic. Because the patient is getting worse you add more drug or another antibiotic. Immunity is considered as an antibiotic activity but without resistance. But you should understand that in many chronic infections, for instance in tuberculosis, mycobacteria are evading the immune response by the formation and evolution of the granuloma, which in a way is mimicking 'resistance to immunity'. This is something which should also be considered in biofilm-producing chronic infections.

Levin: You are quite right. In this model we are indeed assuming that the immune system is behaving like an antibiotic, the concentration of which will increase with the density of the pathogen. In the case of tuberculosis, we are assuming that in patients with this disease in its acute form, frank tuberculosis, the infection is out of the control of the host defences and the bacteria are growing without bounds. Chemotherapy is essential to control the infection. As in our other models, chemotherapy can bring the population of sensitive *M. tuberculosis* down to below a lethal density. At the total number of cells considered, clones resistant to single antibiotics are almost certainly present. The primary focus of the analysis of our models is on the conditions under which bacteria resistant to more than one of the treating antibiotics will arise and the role of tissue heterogeneity in the sensitivity to different antibiotics in this evolution.

Davies: What is *E. coli* K1 and what kind of infection does it cause in mice?

Levin: It causes a lethal septicaemia, presumably because of the host response to the LPS. The K1 capsule seems to play a role in this process by increasing the survival of the bacteria in the serum and possibly other tissues. High density infections of K1 negative variants of this strain (an 018:K1:H7) are non-lethal. When introduced into the thigh at densities in excess of 10^7, these K1-negative strains grow but disseminate at lower rates than the K1-positive.

Davies: Is *E. coli* K1 particularly virulent in mice?

Levin: Yes, but it's not exactly a natural infection. When we inoculate it at densities of 10^7 into the thighs of mice it proliferates rapidly, disseminates and kills the mouse, usually within 30–40 h. As I said earlier, the K1-negative variant does not kill the mouse even when inoculated at substantially higher densities. The *E. coli* K1-positive strain is responsible for neonatal sepsis in human infants.

Lerner: Does your model depend on the rate of killing by different antibiotics, and also on the rate being dependent on the concentrations?

Levin: Yes. The concentrations of antibiotics are waxing and waning every time you pulse them, so the rate of killing is changing.

Lerner: The rate of killing is concentration-dependent for some antibiotics, such as aminoglycosides and quinolones, but less variable for others, such as β-lactams, at least while the concentration is above the MIC.

Levin: I am sure it varies for all of them, but to different degrees. Whether or not you get below the MIC is a critical point. If in fact you have a way of keeping the antibiotics in all tissues above the MIC, you should clear the infection.

Lerner: Did you play with the kinetics of the antituberculosis drugs? We don't really know how to give these agents optimally; no one has studied this carefully.

Levin: One of the goals of our theoretical studies is to meld the within-host population dynamics of the bacteria and the host defences with the pharmacokinetics and pharmacodynamics of the antibiotics. There is an abundance of wonderful literature on this subject by E. R. Garrett (Garrett & Won 1973) and on the role of tissue heterogeneity in anti-tuberculosis chemotherapy by D. A. Mitchison (1979) that we are relying on for this enterprise. In addition to doing the modelling we are using experimental infections in mice to test the validity of the assumptions behind the construction of these models and their predictions. One of the longer-range goals of this jointly theoretical and empirical enterprise is to develop models that are sufficiently realistic and precise to be of use for designing treatment protocols. It is clear that we are some way from achieving this goal. How far away is not so clear.

Levy: What experimental data are out there to tell you the rates of mutation in mycobacteria? The community is readily accepting the fact that point mutations accumulate in *Mycobacterium*. In the 1950s, when *E. coli* emerged with multidrug resistance it was unacceptable that this could be the result of multiple point mutations. Yet with *M. tuberculosis* we're accepting it. Your model suggests that mutations are sequential but they could be compartmental. What is the evidence that the tuberculosis organism moves from compartment to compartment or tissue to tissue? Resistance emerging in one tissue would then be taken to another tissue. What are the conditions under which the mutations are occurring? Are anaerobic conditions more likely to give you a mutation than aerobic conditions, and are they more likely to occur in the lung than in an abscess or in some other place in the body?

Lipsitch: There were two papers in the early 1970s that measured mutation rates to drug resistance in *M. tuberculosis* (David 1970, David & Newman 1971). They measured the rates of mutation to resistance to streptomycin, rifampin, isoniazid and ethambutol. The mutation rates were in the order of 10^{-7} or 10^{-8} for all drugs except rifampin, which was around 2×10^{-10}. This is a surprisingly low number, an order of magnitude lower than in *E. coli*, although the mutations in both cases are alterations to the *rpoB* gene. It would be interesting to replicate David's (1970) fluctuation test to confirm that very low mutation rate. There has been some discussion of why, in immunocompetent treated patients in whom resistance emerges, isoniazid resistance tends to come first. The usual argument is that it is because the mutation rate is 100 times higher (Nolan et al 1995). One result of our model is that even with such large differences in mutation rates, selection pressures, rather than mutation rates, play the major role in determining which drug resistance arises first.

Levin: Our estimates of the rate of mutation to rifampin resistance in *E. coli* considerably exceed the 10^{-10} figure used for *M. tuberculosis*.

Roberts: TB grows very slowly, and in a lot of cases you still have a lot of bugs around even if you do not have severe disease. We know that mutations can accumulate even when organisms are not actually growing. This may play a role in the development of resistance: in most infections where you get rid of the organisms from the body, the microbes have to start over again accumulating mutations, whereas in TB the organisms often hang around for a long time. Thus, if we believe that what happens in *E. coli* could happen in *Mycobacterium*, we can envisage the development of multiple drug resistance, especially in patients that have been non-compliant.

Cohen: Theoretically you could get compartmentalization during infection by the nature of granuloma formation.

With respect to non-compliance, your model involves non-compliance to both drugs at the same time. What often happens is that patients run out of or stop taking one drug, so there is intermittent exposure to different antibiotics. How would this affect the model?

Levin: Non-compliant individuals taking single drugs could, in fact, be more problematic than those who fail to take any drug at all.

References

Antia R, Levin BR, May RM 1994 Within-host population dynamics and the evolution and maintenance of microparasite virulence. Am Nat 144:457–472

David HL 1970 Probability distribution of drug resistant mutants in unselected populations of *Mycobacterium tuberculosis*. Appl Microbiol 20:810–814

David HL, Newman CM 1971 Some observations on the genetics of isoniazid resistance in the tubercle bacilli. Am Rev Respir Dis 104:508–515

Garrett ER, Won CM 1973 Kinetics and mechanisms of actions of drugs on microorganisms. VII. Quantitative adherence of sulfonamide action on microbial growth to a receptor-site model. J Pharm Sci 56:1576–1585

Mitchison DA 1979 Basic mechanisms of chemotherapy. Chest 76:771–781

Nolan CM, Williams DL, Cave MD et al 1995 Evolution of rifampin resistance in human immunodeficiency virus-associated tuberculosis. Am J Respir Crit Care Med 152:1067–1071

The cost of antibiotic resistance — from the perspective of a bacterium

Richard E. Lenski

Center for Microbial Ecology, Michigan State University, East Lansing, MI 48824, USA

Abstract. The possession of an antibiotic resistance gene clearly benefits a bacterium when the corresponding antibiotic is present. But does the resistant bacterium suffer a cost of resistance (i.e. a reduction in fitness) when the antibiotic is absent? If so, then one strategy to control the spread of resistance would be to suspend the use of a particular antibiotic until resistant genotypes declined to low frequency. Numerous studies have indeed shown that resistant genotypes are less fit than their sensitive counterparts in the absence of antibiotic, indicating a cost of resistance. But there is an important caveat: these studies have put antibiotic resistance genes into naïve bacteria, which have no evolutionary history of association with the resistance genes. An important question, therefore, is whether bacteria can overcome the cost of resistance by evolving adaptations that counteract the harmful side-effects of resistance genes. In fact, several experiments have shown that the cost of antibiotic resistance may be substantially diminished, even eliminated, by evolutionary changes in bacteria over rather short periods of time. As a consequence of this adaptation of bacteria to their resistance genes, it becomes increasingly difficult to eliminate resistant genotypes simply by suspending the use of antibiotics.

1997 Antibiotic resistance: origins, evolution, selection and spread. Wiley, Chichester (Ciba Foundation Symposium 207) p 131–151

Antibiotic-resistant bacteria impose a tremendous economic burden on the human population. In addition to morbidity and mortality caused by failure to cure those individuals who are infected by resistant pathogens, society as a whole must pay for the research and development of new antibiotics to keep pace with continually evolving pathogens. It is clear, therefore, that there are major costs associated with antibiotic resistance from the perspective of human society. But is there any cost associated with antibiotic resistance from the perspective of a bacterium?

In an environment that contains antibiotic, possession of a corresponding resistance gene is clearly beneficial to a bacterium. However, in the absence of antibiotic, resistant genotypes may have growth rates that are lower than their sensitive counterparts. Mutations that confer resistance do so by disrupting some normal physiological process in the cell, thereby causing detrimental side-effects. In the case of plasmid-encoded resistance functions, bacteria must synthesize additional nucleic acids and proteins; this synthesis imposes an energetic burden (DaSilva & Bailey 1986) and the products that are synthesized may also interfere with the cell's physiology (Lenski & Nguyen 1988). Resistant bacteria may therefore be inferior competitors to sensitive genotypes in the absence of antibiotics. If so, then a possible strategy for containing the spread of antibiotic resistance would be to suspend the use of a particular antibiotic until the corresponding resistant genotypes had declined to low frequency.

Figure 1 shows that the efficacy of this strategy depends on the cost of resistance from the perspective of the bacterium. Assuming that some sensitive genotypes have survived antibiotic treatment (or that they colonized after the treatment ended), the amount of time that would be required to reduce the abundance of resistant bacteria to a specified low level is inversely proportional to the cost of resistance. For example, it takes 10 times as long to eliminate a population of resistant bacteria when the cost of resistance is only 1% compared with when the cost of resistance is 10%. Thus, the efficacy of controlling the spread of antibiotic resistance by suspending antibiotic treatment is critically dependent on the relative fitness of resistant and sensitive genotypes.

In the following sections, I review several experiments that have sought to measure the costs of antibiotic resistance from the perspective of bacteria. The major findings are twofold. On the one hand, it is true that resistant bacteria often are inferior competitors to their sensitive counterparts in the absence of antibiotic. On the other hand, the costs of antibiotic resistance to bacteria are subject to evolutionary change, and so they tend to be reduced over time by natural selection. Unfortunately, this trend implies that it will become increasingly difficult over time to control the spread of resistant strains simply by suspending the usage of a particular antibiotic.

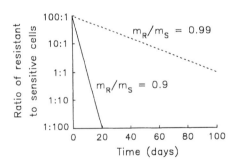

FIG. 1.   Effect of the cost of resistance on the persistence of antibiotic-resistant bacteria after the antibiotic is discontinued. Consider a mixture of resistant and sensitive bacteria with abundances of R and S, respectively. The relative abundance of resistant and sensitive cells over time, t, is governed by the equation: $\ln[R(t)/S(t)] = \ln[R(0)/S(0)] - (m_S - m_R)t$, where m_S and m_R are the growth rates (net of cell death) of sensitive and resistant cells, respectively, in the absence of antibiotic. In the figure, m_S is set at 4.6 per day, and m_R is expressed as a percentage of m_S.

Consensus findings indicate a cost to resistance

Many studies have shown that resistant genotypes are less fit than their sensitive progenitors in antibiotic-free medium. The essential element of these studies involves competition between sensitive and resistant genotypes that are otherwise isogenic (Fig. 2). Some of these studies have demonstrated costs associated with carriage of plasmids and expression of plasmid-encoded resistance functions (e.g. Zünd & Lebek 1980), whereas other studies have demonstrated side-effects of resistance mutations that impair growth (e.g. Jin & Gross 1989).

I am not aware of a systematic review of these studies, perhaps because the results are often included in papers dealing with other topics and because the conclusion seems so obvious. None the less, I am confident that the literature contains tens, if not hundreds, of cases in which resistance has been shown to reduce bacterial competitiveness in the absence of antibiotic. (Several of these cases will be discussed below when we examine the evolutionary modification of the costs of resistance.) The literature also probably contains some cases in which there was no discernible cost of antibiotic resistance. Perhaps these results reflect a real absence of a cost, or perhaps they simply indicate that the cost was too small to be seen given the experimental resolution. For example, Nguyen et al (1989) observed a large and significant cost due to constitutive expression of a plasmid-encoded tetracycline resistance function in *Escherichia coli*, but they could not measure any significant cost for an inducible resistance function beyond a small cost associated with carriage of the plasmid vector itself. Evidently, repression of a resistance function can be quite effective in avoiding the cost of resistance in an antibiotic-free environment.

In contrast to the numerous studies that have measured a cost associated with antibiotic resistance, I know of only one study in which a resistance function was

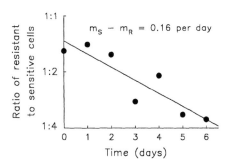

FIG. 2.   Illustration of a competition experiment to measure the cost of antibiotic resistance in the absence of antibiotic (redrawn from Lenski et al 1994). Symbols show the relative abundance of two E. *coli* genotypes, one of which carries a plasmid that encodes antibiotic resistance. In the experiment, the net growth rate of sensitive cells, m_S, was about 4.6 per day, while the difference in growth rates between sensitive and resistant cells, $m_S - m_R$, was estimated by linear regression to be 0.16 per day. The plasmid evidently reduces its host's fitness relative to the plasmid-free competitor.

shown to confer an immediate (see below) selective advantage even in the absence of antibiotic. Blot et al (1991) showed that a Tn*5*-encoded bleomycin-resistance gene enhanced the survival of *E. coli* during prolonged starvation, even though no antibiotic was present in the medium. Bleomycin causes damage to DNA, and DNA damage may also occur during prolonged starvation. The gene product that is responsible for bleomycin resistance is thought to play some role in DNA repair, which may explain its beneficial effect during prolonged starvation.

But there is a caveat

The evidence summarized in the preceding section indicates that antibiotic-resistant bacteria are usually at a competitive disadvantage relative to their sensitive counterparts when there is no antibiotic present in the environment. However, there is an important qualification to this conclusion. That is, these studies have been performed by putting an antibiotic-resistance gene (either a plasmid-encoded function or a chromosomal mutation) into a 'naïve' bacterium, one which has no evolutionary history of association with that resistance gene. An important question, therefore, is whether the cost of resistance can be reduced or even eliminated by allowing the bacterium to adapt to the resistance gene. I will now review several experimental studies that sought to address this issue.

Evolutionary reductions in the cost of plasmid-encoded antibiotic resistance

Plasmid pACYC184 encodes resistance to two antibiotics, tetracycline and chloramphenicol. Bouma & Lenski (1988) transformed a laboratory strain of *E. coli* with pACYC184, and they showed that the plasmid-bearing construct was an inferior competitor relative to its plasmid-free counterpart in a glucose-minimal medium without antibiotic (Fig. 3A). The bacterial strain that they used had no history of association with pACYC184, and so they sought to determine if the cost of plasmid carriage could be reduced by evolutionary changes in either the host or the plasmid. To that end, Bouma & Lenski propagated the plasmid–host association for 500 generations (75 d) in the same glucose-minimal medium, except now supplemented with chloramphenicol. (The supplemental antibiotic was necessary to prevent spontaneous plasmid-free segregants from out-competing the plasmid-bearing cells, which would have defeated the purpose of the experiment.)

At the end of 500 generations, Bouma & Lenski (1988) isolated a spontaneous plasmid-free segregant of the evolved bacterial host. They then transformed each of the ancestral and evolved hosts with both the ancestral and evolved plasmids, giving them four genotypes: B_0/P_0, B_0/P_{500}, B_{500}/P_0, and B_{500}/P_{500}, where B and P denote the bacteria and plasmid, respectively, and subscripts 0 and 500 indicate the ancestral (naïve) and evolved forms, respectively. Each of these genotypes was allowed to compete against a genetically marked variant of B_0/P_0 in the same medium used during the 500 generations of experimental evolution. These competition

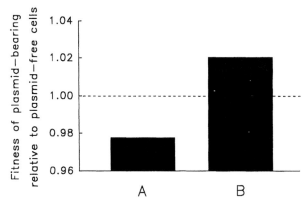

FIG. 3. Effects of pACYC184 on the fitness of ancestral and evolved E. *coli* hosts, in the absence of antibiotic (summary of data from Lenski et al 1994). B_0 denotes the ancestral genotype, and B_{500} is a genotype that evolved with pACYC184 for 500 generations. (A) Fitness of B_0/pACYC184 versus its plasmid-free counterpart, B_0. (B) Fitness of B_{500}/pACYC184 versus its plasmid-free counterpart, B_{500}. The values shown in (A) and (B) are the means of 30 replicate competition experiments. The costs and benefits of plasmid carriage for the ancestral and evolved genotypes, respectively, are highly significant ($P < 0.001$).

experiments indicated that genetic adaptation had occurred in the bacterial chromosome, but not in the plasmid. That is, B_{500} was competitively superior to B_0, and this advantage was unaffected by the plasmid's evolutionary history (or lack thereof). These competition experiments demonstrated that the bacteria had adapted evolutionarily, but they did not show whether the bacteria had adapted to the plasmid, to the culture medium, or to some combination of the two.

To determine whether the bacteria had adapted to the plasmid, Bouma & Lenski (1988) performed competition experiments in antibiotic-free medium between the evolved bacteria with and without the ancestral plasmid (i.e. B_{500}/P_0 versus B_{500}). If the bacterial host had adapted specifically to the plasmid, then the cost of carriage should be lower in the evolved bacteria than in the ancestor. To their surprise, Bouma & Lenski found that the evolved plasmid-bearing bacteria had a competitive advantage relative to the evolved plasmid-free bacteria even in the absence of antibiotic (Fig. 3B). Thus, not only had the cost of plasmid carriage been eliminated, but the plasmid was actually beneficial to the bacteria that had evolved with the plasmid present.

Lenski et al (1994) sought to identify what aspect of the plasmid was beneficial to the evolved bacterial host, but not to its naïve ancestor. They constructed a series of new plasmids from pACYC184 in which they deleted either the chloramphenicol or tetracycline resistance functions. Resistance to chloramphenicol occurs by the enzymic acetylation of the antibiotic, which renders it inactive. Resistance to tetracycline involves active efflux of the antibiotic using a transmembrane protein. They showed that expression of the chloramphenicol resistance function imposed a significant cost for both the naïve and evolved host bacteria. However, expression of

TABLE 1 Expression of tetracycline resistance is beneficial to an *E. coli* host that evolved with plasmid pACYC184

Plasmid	Cm	Tc	Naïve Host	Evolved Host
pACYC184	R	R	—	+
pMP10	S	R	0	++
pMP11	S	R	0	++
pSCS1	R	S	—	—
pSCS13	R	S	—	—

Data from Lenski et al (1994). Cm, chloramphenicol; Tc, tetracycline; R, resistant; S, sensitive. Plasmids pMP10 and pMP11 have deletions in the gene for chloramphenicol resistance. Plasmids pSCS1 and pSCS13 have deletions in the gene for tetracycline resistance. The last two columns indicate the effect of plasmid carriage on the fitness of naïve and evolved bacterial hosts, in the absence of antibiotic. —, significant cost; 0, no significant effect; +, significant benefit; ++, significantly larger benefit.

the tetracycline resistance function was actually beneficial to the evolved bacteria (but not to the naïve ancestor) in the absence of antibiotic. That is, an evolved host which carries a plasmid that expresses tetracycline resistance is competitively superior to its plasmid-free counterpart, whereas an evolved host which carries a plasmid that does not express tetracycline resistance is less fit than its plasmid-free counterpart (Table 1).

Although the physiological basis of this effect is not yet fully understood, this study shows clearly that the cost of plasmid-encoded antibiotic resistance can be reduced or even eliminated by natural selection. When pACYC184 was first introduced into the naïve bacterium, it was lost from the population in the absence of antibiotic as spontaneous plasmid-free segregants competitively excluded the plasmid-bearing cells. But as a consequence of the evolutionary adaptation of the bacteria to the plasmid, plasmid-free segregants no longer have a competitive advantage and the plasmid-encoded antibiotic resistance is stably maintained.

In a conceptually similar study, Modi & Adams (1991) examined the coevolution of *E. coli* and a derivative of plasmid pBR322 that encodes resistance to ampicillin and tetracycline. After about 800 generations, they found that the cost of plasmid carriage to the bacterial host had been significantly reduced, although it was not entirely eliminated in this case. They also showed that genetic changes in both the bacterial and plasmid genomes contributed to the reduced cost of plasmid carriage. As with the previous study, Modi & Adams' results indicate that it may become much more difficult to eliminate antibiotic resistance after bacteria and plasmids have had an evolutionary history of association.

Evolutionary reductions in the cost of chromosomal mutations that confer antibiotic resistance

The finding that the cost of antibiotic resistance can be reduced is not restricted to plasmid-encoded resistance. In a recent study, Schrag & Perrot (1996) examined mutations in the *rpsL* gene of *E. coli* that confer resistance to streptomycin. In the absence of antibiotic, cells that carry these mutations are handicapped in competition with otherwise isogenic cells that are sensitive to streptomycin. The streptomycin-resistant mutants have altered ribosomes and a lower rate of peptide-chain elongation, which may account for the cost of resistance. Schrag & Perrot (1996) also sought to determine if the cost of antibiotic resistance could be reduced by allowing the bacteria to evolve. After less than 200 generations of evolution in the absence of antibiotic, they found that the cost of resistance was substantially reduced. This cost-reduction was achieved without any significant change in the level of streptomycin resistance. Schrag & Perrot further demonstrated that this cost-reduction was achieved by secondary mutations outside of the *rpsL* gene, and that these secondary mutations restored the rate of peptide-chain elongation to a level close to that of the streptomycin-sensitive progenitor (Fig. 4). Thus, evolving populations of bacteria tend to compensate for the deleterious side-effects of their resistance genes, including mutations as well as plasmid-encoded functions.

Cohan et al (1994) examined the cost of resistance to rifampicin in *Bacillus subtilis*. Mutations that confer resistance to rifampicin occur in the *rpoB* gene, which encodes the β-subunit of the RNA polymerase, and these mutations tend to reduce the competitive fitness of the bacteria in the absence of antibiotic. However, Cohan et al demonstrated that the magnitude of this cost was highly variable depending on the specific mutation to rifampicin resistance as well as the particular strain of *B. subtilis* into which a mutation was transformed. (The cost of resistance did not correlate with the level of rifampicin resistance, which was high for all combinations of resistance alleles and genetic backgrounds.) This study therefore implies two distinct mechanisms by which the cost of resistance can be ameliorated. First, selection among resistance alleles will favour those which impose the lowest costs. Second,

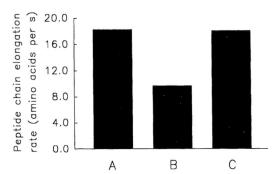

FIG. 4.   Rates of peptide chain elongation in *E. coli* that are sensitive and resistant to streptomycin (summary of data from Schrag & Perrot 1996). (A) Ancestral sensitive genotype. (B) Average of two resistant genotypes. (C) Average of four resistant genotypes after 180 generations of evolutionary cost-reduction. The difference between (A) and (B) is statistically significant, whereas the difference between (A) and (C) is not.

selection among genetic backgrounds will favour those which are subject to the lowest costs. As a consequence of selection, the cost of resistance to rifampicin should become progressively reduced over time, as only the most fit combinations of resistance alleles and genetic backgrounds will prevail in competition.

Do similar phenomena occur in nature?

The experiments reviewed above (showing both the cost of resistance and its evolutionary reduction) were all performed in the laboratory, under highly simplified conditions. There is every reason to believe, however, that similar phenomena occur in nature. The lack of direct evidence for these phenomena reflects the fact that it would be very difficult in a natural setting to perform the rigorous manipulative experiments that are necessary to quantify subtle differences in competitive fitness. None the less, there is some suggestive evidence from nature for evolutionary reductions in the cost of antibiotic resistance.

For example, *Neisseria gonorrhoeae* was considered for many years to be universally susceptible to penicillin and its derivatives such as ampicillin. In 1976, however, resistant strains that produced β-lactamase were detected, and this resistance was plasmid-encoded. According to Roberts et al (1977), the resistance plasmids that were first isolated from *N. gonorrhoeae* were very unstable, but within a few months the resistance plasmids that were sampled had become more stable. A possible explanation for this increased stability is an evolutionary reduction in the cost of antibiotic resistance, because plasmid stability is affected by even small differences in the growth rates of plasmid-bearing cells and plasmid-free segregants (Cooper et al 1987, Lenski & Bouma 1987). Had some other antibiotic been used temporarily to treat gonorrhoea when resistance to ampicillin was first detected, then resistance might have rapidly disappeared from the *N. gonorrhoeae* population; ampicillin could then have been used for many more years.

Evolutionary reductions in the cost of resistance have also been suggested as possible explanations for the surprising persistence of resistance to tetracycline and streptomycin (Smith 1975, Johnson & Adams 1992, Sundin & Bender 1996). The possible role of evolutionary cost-reduction in extending the persistence of antibiotic-resistance genes in nature deserves careful further study.

Evolutionary cost-reduction is not restricted to antibiotic resistance

The proliferation of antibiotic-resistant bacteria provides an especially dramatic example of biological evolution because of its rapidity as well as its medical importance. However, the evolution of resistance functions, the costs associated with resistance functions and the subsequent amelioration of these costs can be seen in other circumstances as well. For example, populations of bacteria readily adapt to the presence of virulent phages in their environment by mutations that prevent phage adsorption (e.g. Lenski & Levin 1985). In the absence of phage, however, resistant genotypes are usually inferior competitors to their sensitive counterparts. Lenski (1988) allowed populations of phage T4-resistant *E. coli* to evolve for 400 generations (60 d) in the absence of phage. Despite a substantial cost of resistance, the evolving bacterial populations did not revert to sensitivity (probably because the mutations were deletions that could not be easily reverted). Instead, other mutations were selected in the evolving bacterial populations that reduced the cost of resistance by about 50%, and they did so without diminishing the extent of resistance itself.

Evolutionary reductions in the cost of resistance functions are also not limited to bacteria. McKenzie et al (1982) describe a compelling example of this phenomenon in an insect pest. For about ten years, the insecticide diazinon was used successfully to control the Australian sheep blowfly, *Lucilia cuprina*. A mutation that conferred resistance eventually appeared and diazinon-resistant flies subsequently became prevalent. At first, the resistant flies developed more slowly and had reduced survival relative to their sensitive progenitors in the absence of insecticide, indicating a cost of resistance. After a few more years of continued usage of diazinon, however, a second mutation appeared in the fly population that eliminated the cost of resistance. Diazinon-resistant flies that had this second mutation were as fit as sensitive flies, even in the absence of diazinon. Thus, the opportunity to control the spread of resistance by temporarily suspending the use of diazinon was lost.

It should be clear from these additional examples in other systems that a reduction in the cost of antibiotic resistance is not some mysterious or unexpected phenomenon. Instead, cost-reduction is a simple and general manifestation of the tendency for organisms to undergo genetic adaptation by natural selection. Just as organisms may adapt to overcome adverse aspects of their external environment (e.g. by becoming resistant to antibiotics), so too may they adapt to overcome adverse aspects of their internal physiology (e.g. by reducing harmful side-effects of resistance).

Conclusions

(1) The sensitivity of bacterial pathogens to antibiotics can be viewed as a natural resource, one which has tremendous value to the human population. Unfortunately, much of this resource has already been depleted in the last half-century, as a consequence of the evolution of pathogens that are resistant to antibiotics.

(2) In principle, antibiotic sensitivity is a renewable resource. If there is a cost of resistance to bacteria, then sensitivity may be renewed by temporarily suspending the use of an antibiotic to which resistance has emerged, thereby allowing sensitive genotypes to competitively displace their resistant counterparts.

(3) However, after evolving resistance to antibiotics, bacteria may then adapt to the deleterious side-effects and other costs of resistance genes. Therefore, with continued use of an antibiotic after the emergence of resistant genotypes, it may become increasingly difficult to renew sensitivity.

Acknowledgements

I wish to thank S. Levy and the Ciba Foundation for organizing a stimulating meeting on this very important topic. I would also like to thank the many colleagues who have discussed these ideas with me and contributed to the research reviewed here. My research is currently supported by a grant from the US National Science Foundation (DEB-9421237).

References

Blot M, Meyer J, Arber W 1991 Bleomycin-resistance gene derived from transposon Tn5 confers selective advantage to *Escherichia coli* K-12. Proc Natl Acad Sci USA 88:9112–9116

Bouma JE, Lenski RE 1988 Evolution of a bacteria/plasmid association. Nature 335:351–352

Cohan FM, King EC, Zawadzki P 1994 Amelioration of the deleterious pleiotropic effects of an adaptive mutation in *Bacillus subtilis*. Evolution 48:81–95

Cooper NS, Brown ME, Caulcott CA 1987 A mathematical model for analysing plasmid stability in microorganisms. J Gen Microbiol 133:1871–1880

DaSilva NA, Bailey JE 1986 Theoretical growth yield estimates for recombinant cells. Biotech Bioeng 28:741–746

Jin DJ, Gross CA 1989 Characterization of the pleiotropic phenotypes of rifampin-resistant *rpoB* mutants of *Escherichia coli*. J Bacteriol 171:5229–5231

Johnson R, Adams J 1992 The ecology and evolution of tetracycline resistance. Trends Ecol Evol 7:295–299

Lenski RE 1988 Experimental studies of pleiotropy and epistasis in *Escherichia coli*. II. Compensation for maladaptive effects associated with resistance to virus T4. Evolution 42:433–440

Lenski RE, Bouma JE 1987 Effect of segregation and selection on instability of plasmid pACYC184 in *Escherichia coli* B. J Bacteriol 169:5314–5316

Lenski RE, Levin BR 1985 Constraints on the coevolution of bacteria and virulent phage: a model, some experiments, and predictions for natural communities. Am Nat 125:585–602

Lenski RE, Nguyen TT 1988 Stability of recombinant DNA and its effects on fitness. Trends Ecol Evol (suppl) 3:18–20

Lenski RE, Simpson SC, Nguyen TT 1994 Genetic analysis of a plasmid-encoded, host genotype-specific enhancement of bacterial fitness. J Bacteriol 176:3140–3147

McKenzie JA, Whitten MJ, Adena MA 1982 The effect of genetic background on the fitness of the diazinon resistance genotypes of the Australian sheep blowfly, *Lucilia cuprina*. Heredity 49:1–9

Modi RI, Adams J 1991 Coevolution in bacteria-plasmid populations. Evolution 45:656–667

Nguyen TNM, Phan QG, Duong LP, Bertrand KP, Lenski RE 1989 Effects of carriage and expression of the Tn10 tetracycline-resistance operon on the fitness of *Escherichia coli* K12. Mol Biol Evol 6:213–225

Roberts M, Elwell LP, Falkow S 1977 Molecular characterization of two β-lactamase-specifying plasmids isolated from *Neisseria gonorrhoeae*. J Bacteriol 131:557–563

Schrag SJ, Perrot V 1996 Reducing antibiotic resistance. Nature 381:120–121

Smith HW 1975 Persistence of tetracycline resistance in pig *E. coli*. Nature 258:628–630

Sundin GW, Bender CL 1996 Dissemination of the *strA-strB* streptomycin-resistance genes among commensal and pathogenic bacteria from humans, animals, and plants. Mol Ecol 5:133–143

Zünd P, Lebek G 1980 Generation time-prolonging R plasmids: correlation between increases in the generation time of *Escherichia coli* caused by R plasmids and their molecular size. Plasmid 3:65–69

DISCUSSION

Roberts: With regard to our study on penicillin-resistant *Neisseria gonorrhoeae* you mentioned (Roberts et al 1977), originally there were two β-lactamase plasmids that looked similar, the 4.4 mDa and the 3.2 mDa plasmid. The smaller 3.2 mDa one conferred a lower MIC. We found that the 4.4 mDa, originally from Asia, was quite stable without antibiotic present. On the other hand, we lost the 3.2 mDa plasmid in 99% of the cells in the absence of the selecting antibiotic in broth, which made it somewhat more difficult to isolate. Shortly thereafter, we started getting isolates from Africa in which the 3.2 mDa plasmids didn't display this phenomenon: we could maintain 50%–70% of the cells with the plasmid. Twenty years down the road these plasmids have spread almost everywhere. If bacteria containing them are grown without the selecting antibiotic, 10–15% may be lost, but nowhere like what we saw originally. In most cases the plasmid sequences are not significantly different, so it's certainly not a plasmid phenomenon. Rather, the organisms have become adapted to surviving with this multicopy plasmid.

Levin: Does the plasmid change the host's fitness or its segregation rate? Have you ever done any analysis to ascertain which component is changing?

Roberts: No. We studied this primarily because we couldn't isolate the plasmid and we wanted to understand why. We did a time-course on how many cells still had the plasmid versus susceptibility.

Lenski: Either type of change would cause persistence of the resistance gene for a longer period. While it would be interesting to know whether there was a change in the plasmid's segregation rate or the effect of plasmid carriage on host fitness, the broader point remains the same. That is, antibiotic resistance was stabilized over time.

Baquero: Do you expect that non-transmissible plasmids will have a different type of behaviour in causing the acquisition of compensating mutations than transmissible plasmids?

Lenski: That is an interesting question. Some mathematical models suggest that the degree to which these elements are moving from host to host (horizontal transmission) versus dividing alongside the host (vertical transmission) is likely to affect some of these properties. The theoretical expectation is that plasmids that are transmitted only vertically, such as non-conjugative plasmids, are going to be under greater pressure to reduce their harmful effects on bacteria. The other way to put this is that there is a greater opportunity for co-adaptation of the host to non-conjugative plasmids than to plasmids that make their living by moving around between different bacterial strains via conjugation.

Baquero: Thus to a certain extent the non-transmissible plasmids are having a pathogenic effect on bacteria.

Lenski: If we move from looking at this from the perspective of the bacterium to that of the plasmids, they also have a lot of evolutionary flexibility. One would expect that during the early phase of an epidemic (where I'm now defining the epidemic by the spread of the resistance gene), transmissibility is going to be highly advantageous to the plasmid. However, as the bacterial population in which a plasmid is found becomes dominated by cells that are already carrying the plasmid, the plasmid would tend to get rid of its conjugative functions. That is because these functions no longer help the plasmid to spread, and yet they slow down the growth of their bacterial hosts (Levin 1980, Turner 1995).

Levy: In studies that we performed among wild baboons in Africa, we found only small numbers of large conjugative plasmids in *E. coli* from the faeces of baboons living in the wild whereas we found smaller multicopy plasmids in the *E. coli* from faeces of baboons rummaging among refuse from people (Levy 1986).

Sköld: This adaptability can also be illustrated by chromosomal resistance to sulfonamides. It is relatively easy to select sulfonamide-resistant mutants of *E. coli* grown on plates. If one looks at the target enzyme, dihydropteroate synthase, one amino acid is changed and there is a 150-fold increase in K_i. In this experimental situation, however, the enzyme has paid a price—the K_m is increased 10-fold. This can be compared with a clinical situation. Sulfonamide resistance is very common in *Neisseria meningitidis*, and we have one example of this where the chromosomal gene for dihydropteroate synthase has an insert of serine and glycine, which increases the K_i some 50 times. If you correct that insertion by site-directed mutagenesis, the K_i drops to that of the wild-type enzyme, but the previously normal K_m increases 60-fold. It seems that one or several compensatory mutations have occurred, making this enzyme completely adapted to function optimally both in the presence and absence of sulfonamide.

Davies: Some time ago Zünd & Lebek (1980) isolated a large number of *E. coli* and *Salmonella* strains from the environment and found them to contain many different plasmids, both large and small. When these strains were propagated in liquid medium in the laboratory, the small plasmids were lost from the cells but the large plasmids (in general) were stably maintained. Loss of the small plasmids was associated with an increase in growth rate of the bacteria. I don't think anyone has been able to interpret these experiments.

With respect to the studies of streptomycin resistance, it is my understanding that many of the streptomycin resistance mutations mapped to *rpsL* were phenotypically streptomycin dependent or streptomycin stimulated, although very weakly so. Were the streptomycin resistant strains that you described examined in the presence of low or high concentrations of streptomycin? There are many different phenotypes found as a result of *rpsL* mutations and weak dependence could be followed by the appearance of compensatory mutations.

Levin: The *rpsL* mutants studied by the two postdocs in my lab, Stephanie Schrag and Veronique Perrot, were not streptomycin dependent (Schrag & Perrot 1996). Both were mutants in the 42nd codon of *rpsL*, with ACA and AAC instead of the wild-type AAA. The former had a 14% growth rate disadvantage relative to the wild-type and the latter a 19% fitness disadvantage, estimates similar to those made much earlier for *E. coli* K12. Stephanie and Veronique were using the same K1-negative variant of *E. coli*, 018:K1:H7, that we were using in our mouse infection studies. After maintaining these streptomycin-resistant strains for 180 generations in serial transfer culture, the dominant clones isolated were resistant to streptomycin but were of substantially greater fitness than their ancestors, albeit not quite as fit as the wild-type streptomycin-sensitive bacteria they were derived from. Moreover, the rate of protein elongation, which was markedly reduced in the *rpsL* mutants, was restored to near wild-type levels, presumably by the second-site mutations which compensated for the fitness cost of the *rpsL* locus. More recently, we obtained an even more ominous result. When the evolved strains carrying the fitness-compensating mutations are made streptomycin sensitive by transducing the *rpsL* gene from an *E. coli* K12 with a wild-type allele, these sensitive transductants have a marked disadvantage relative to the resistant. One interpretation of this is that once the second-site mutations are established in the population at large, an adaptive valley is established and you can't go back to streptomycin sensitive.

Davies: Did you test to see whether that cost was reversed in the presence of low concentrations of streptomycin?

Levin: Stephanie and Veronique did their competition experiments in glucose-limited minimal medium without streptomycin or other antibiotics.

Davies: Streptomycin-dependent phenotypes vary enormously. You can get a resistant strain that is dependent on 10 μg/ml of streptomycin or a strain dependent on a 1 μg/ml streptomycin. My point is that the second mutation, which is the compensatory mutation, could alter ribosomal proteins S4 or S5, which are known to alleviate streptomycin dependence and thus re-establish normal growth in the absence of the drug.

Levin: The compensatory mutation didn't re-establish normal growth. The highest fitness acquired by the second-site mutation was about 4% less than that of wild-type *rpsL*.

Davies: It sounds as if an alteration in another ribosomal protein was selected.

Levin: I agree. A likely reason that you can't go back is that to compensate for the fitness costs of the *rpsL* mutation, the configuration of the ribosome was changed by a second site mutation at another ribosomal protein locus. With that alteration, a ribosome with a wild-type *rpsL*-encoded protein would be even less effective than one with the streptomycin-resistant *rpsL*.

Retrospective observations are also consistent with this 'can't go back again' interpretation. Despite all of the changes Richard Lenski and his colleagues observed in the 10 000 generation evolution studies in streptomycin-free medium (e.g. Travisano et al 1995), the strain of *E. coli* B they were using remained *rpsL* due to an ACA mutation at the 42nd codon. When we replaced the streptomycin-resistant *rpsL* locus with that of a sensitive *E. coli* B ancestor of the strain that Richard and his collaborators used, the streptomycin-sensitive strain was at a disadvantage relative to the resistant.

Davies: Some *E. coli* strains show differential phenotypic expression of *str* alleles. For example, a *strD* mutation from *E. coli* K12 was expressed as sensitive in *E. coli* C (Luzatto et al 1968)!

Levin: It would be interesting to see how the ribosomes of *E. coli* C and *E. coli* K12 or *E. coli* B differ.

Lenski: The phenomenon of compensation for the cost of resistance to streptomycin may involve some of the same mutations that are involved in streptomycin dependence. However, its evolutionary implications for managing antibiotic resistance are exactly the opposite. Streptomycin dependence would suggest that the bacteria become dependent on the antibiotic, so that in the absence of it they're going to disappear very quickly. By contrast, compensation makes the resistant bacteria more competitive in the absence of antibiotic, so that they will disappear only slowly if at all.

Lipsitch: With reference to the question of whether you can bring the normal flora back and have some sort of competition, one difference between yours and Schrag & Perrot's (1996) experiments is that in their experiments a cost of resistance was maintained even after the evolution of compensatory mutations. There weren't any sensitive strains with the unevolved background, without compensation around for the compensated, resistant strains to compete with. In your experiments there's still some benefit in having the evolved resistance genes even against the old unevolved strains.

Lenski: You are correct in pointing out this difference. In our study (Bouma & Lenski 1988), the evolved resistant bacteria have a selective advantage not only relative to sensitive revertants but also relative to the sensitive progenitor. In the study by Schrag & Perrot (1996; also B. R. Levin, personal communication), however, it seems the evolved resistant bacteria have an advantage relative to sensitive revertants, but not relative to the sensitive progenitor. But even in the latter case, the disadvantage of the evolved resistant bacteria relative to the sensitive progenitor has been substantially reduced. The important and general result is that natural selection will lead to the eventual integration of the resistance mechanism into the overall physiology of the organism. Even if selection cannot get rid of the entire cost of resistance, this phenomenon has important epidemiological consequences. For example, if the cost of resistance is reduced by half, then that will double the time that one must wait to restore a given level of sensitivity after the use of a particular antibiotic is suspended.

Summers: The concepts Richard Lenski has introduced might explain why the ultraviolet resistance determinant *umu* is frequently found on large conjugative plasmids.

I was intrigued that in your pACYC184 experiments, you found that Tet was favoured over chloramphenicol. Is Tet always favoured?

Lenski: Everything that I discussed in my paper was based on a single replication of the evolution experiment. We have now run the evolution experiment six independent times, and we also had control populations where plasmid-free bacteria evolved in the absence of antibiotic for the same number of generations (R. E. Lenski, unpublished results).

Summers: Was it always one antibiotic?

Lenski: Yes, chloramphenicol was used in each replication to ensure retention of the plasmid, and yet in each case the bacteria evolved the dependence on expression of the tetracycline-resistance function. That is, in all six replications of the experiment, the evolved genotypes that were resistant to tetracycline would out-compete sensitive derivatives in the absence of the antibiotic. This change was never observed in any of the derived genotypes that had evolved without the plasmid. So it seems that there is something that predisposes the bacteria that we used to take advantage of the tetracycline-resistance function.

Summers: What is the control of Tet in that particular construct?

Lenski: Tetracycline resistance is constitutively expressed in the plasmid pACYC184. There have been several studies that show a cost of tetracycline resistance in some strains (Nguyen et al 1989 and references therein), and that makes our result even more surprising. However, we have created heterologous plasmids that are pBR322 derivatives. These constructs are also beneficial to the evolved bacteria in our experiment only when they express the Tet function (Lenski et al 1994). Thus, it really is expression of tetracycline resistance that confers this unexpected advantage to the bacteria in the absence of any antibiotic.

Levy: Have you tried this experiment in different media?

Lenski: No, we have just used a minimal medium supplemented with glucose.

Levy: I ask this question because we wonder what other things the Tet determinant might be doing. The Tet L determinant in *Bacillus subtilis* appears also to act as an Na^+/H^+ antiport system (Cheng et al 1996). You might see different effects with a different medium.

Cohen: It might also be interesting to examine some of the currently circulating strains in similar experiments. *Salmonella* and *Shigella* strains very commonly have high frequencies of resistance to tetracycline and streptomycin. It would be fascinating to see if those strains maintain those resistances because of the persistent selective pressure of antibiotics in the environment, or because these strains now have some dependency or other biochemical advantage from the presence of these markers.

Lenski: I agree that this is a very interesting and important question, and we are planning some experiments of the following sort. Dr Valeria Souza, at the Universidad Nacional Autonóma de México, has amassed a large collection of *E. coli* from various settings. Some of these strains are sensitive to tetracycline, for example, whereas other strains carry plasmids that confer resistance. Our plan is to move plasmids from one genetic background (or strain) to the others, and then measure the growth rates of otherwise isogenic plasmid-bearing and plasmid-free cells to determine the cost of plasmid carriage. If the phenomenon of compensation has occurred in nature, then we might see that the cost of plasmid carriage is systematically lower in those strains that have a history of association with the plasmid.

Huovinen: We are talking about resistance genes carried on plasmids; when is it wise for bacteria to transfer these genes to their chromosome?

Levin: I don't know when it would be 'wise' for bacteria to transfer genes from a plasmid to the chromosome or do anything else for that matter. Experimentally, we can select for the transfer of a resistance-encoding transposon from a plasmid to the chromosome by using a plasmid that doesn't replicate and select for that resistance gene. I expect this would also hold when the plasmid has a high rate of vegetative segregation and bacteria are under positive selection of a gene on that plasmid (Condit & Levin 1990). The general question you are asking of when bacterial genes are maintained on accessory elements rather than chromosomes is, to my mind, one of the most interesting yet-to-be answered questions in bacterial evolution.

Levy: Is there a selective pressure to get rid of the plasmid and yet save the tetracycline resistance? In your experiments, Richard, the Tet resistance determinant was important; it did not appear to be the plasmid. What would happen if you put Tn*10* on the chromosome?

Lenski: That's an interesting point. The only problem with that experiment is that one would be introducing an uncontrolled dosage effect, because tetracycline-resistance is expressed constitutively in the strains that we studied. But all else being equal, I agree that the evolved bacteria should benefit from having the resistance determinant on their chromosome, in order to avoid the other costs associated with the rest of plasmid.

Spratt: In the hospital environment, there is so much antibiotic usage that resistant bacteria could survive even if there was a cost. Out in the community where there is much less antibiotic use, there are examples where there's a high level of resistance in pathogens. Do you think that in the community resistant bacteria could survive if there was a cost of resistance? What antibiotic usage in the community would you require to be able to maintain resistant organisms in the face of such a cost?

Lenski: I can't answer that question quantitatively. There's a balance between the forces pushing populations towards resistance versus sensitivity, and that balance is going to differ between hospitals and the community. In principle, bacteria will probably maintain at least some resistance as long as there is even just a little bit of antibiotic selection. My main point is that the nature of the balance itself is changed the longer antibiotic selection is maintained.

Levy: There is likely a cost of resistance, even if it is small. Eventually all that matters is that the susceptible strains have an advantage and can come back. Let's keep them sufficiently numerous so that they come back rapidly. Given enough time, the cost of resistance diminishes, as we cause evolution to select those which are more fit. Consequently, the return to a susceptible flora is going to become increasingly more difficult. I can remember times when we worried about losing plasmids from clinical isolates. I don't hear much about natural plasmid instability now.

Roberts: I can give you another example with *Neisseria gonorrhoeae* where Tet M is carried on a conjugative plasmid and you can't get rid of it, so it is very stable. This was true from the first isolate to the present. Some Gram-negatives have plasmid-associated virulence factors. Now we're starting to see one plasmid with both virulence factors and antibiotic resistance, which certainly changes the equation because that plasmid makes them a better pathogen. There it is a distinct advantage for them because they're being selected for virulence functions and not for the antibiotic resistances.

Piddock: In the pre-licensing days of fluoroquinolones, a lot of people were trying to select laboratory mutants to try and predict what sort of clinical problems might arise. There were several notables in the mid 1980s, stating that clinical resistance to quinolones will not occur because of the difficulty of selecting mutants, and those mutants that were selected grew poorly and lacked various virulence factors (Dalhoff & Doring 1985, Crumplin 1986). This has not translated to the clinical situation. After listening to the last two presentations, I wonder whether we have co-selected for mutations in other genes along with antibiotic resistance. Along with low level resistance as an intermediate we probably have another mutation that allows these virulence markers to still be expressed and not be lost.

Levy: To push that further, it may not be virulence but it may be environmental competitiveness or fitness which is co-selected.

Piddock: But the early work was specifically looking at the expression of virulence markers. There was clearly a loss of them, which hasn't translated to the clinical situation at all.

Davies: I'd like to ask the infectious disease specialists about the cycling of antibiotics in hospitals. Suppose that use of a particular antibiotic is stopped for a certain period. The resistant population diminishes but it never goes away, and when the antibiotic is used again the resistance comes back. Have there been cases where this strategy has actually been effective?

Noble: About 30 years ago in this country Mary Barber was able to restrict the use of antibiotics in an entire hospital, with a reduction in resistant strains (Barber et al 1960). One of the other observations we made in the past was that when patients were discharged carrying a hospital strain and re-admitted perhaps two years later, they had their own domestic strains back again. I don't think that is true nowadays, but I haven't seen any recent documentation.

Bush: There's an interesting observation concerning ceftazidime-resistant *Klebsiella* in the Flushing NY hospital. My laboratory received 12 representative isolates. After several passages of cells we lost the β-lactamase gene responsible for ceftazidime resistance in at least four of these. In the hospital they ceased to use ceftazidime, as one would do in a cycling program situation, and by cutting down ceftazidime use, the incidence of the ceftazidime-resistant *Klebsiella strains* went down considerably, probably due to the loss of the TEM-24 β-lactamase gene as in the laboratory. However, they then started using imipenem and, as a result, began to identify imipenem-resistant *Acinetobacter* (Urban et al 1993), so recycling can simply replace one problem with another.

Baquero: In some areas in the world we have seen that stopping the use of tetracycline or chloramphenicol, for instance, causes the resistance to go down very slowly. For example, *Streptococcus pneumoniae* resistance in Spain halved over 10–15 years.

Giamarellou: To make a rationally based decision about cycling antibiotics it is necessary for one to know the mechanism underlying the resistance in a particular hospital. If, for instance, I have a population of *Enterobacter* spp. resistant to ceftazidime and third-generation cephalosporins, I would know that it is mediated through chromosomal β-lactamases. In that case a fourth generation cephalosporin that is effective against this type of bacterium could be indicated. But if I was dealing with populations of *Klebsiella* which have on the same plasmid the genes for ceftazidime, trimethoprim, tetracycline and aminoglycoside resistance, then how should the cycling be done?

Summers: In addition to the subtle effects that Richard was describing, there are *Kil* and *Kor* systems on most of the large plasmids which are examples of what Mike Yarmolinsky and others have referred to as plasmid 'addiction' (Lehnherr & Yarmolinsky 1995). Once a cell gets one of these big plasmids its *Kil*/*Kor* genes booby-trap the cell, so that if the cell loses the plasmid, it dies. These large plasmids with such *Kil*/*Kor* systems are major players in terms of plasmid-carried resistances. Such systems influence persistence of resistance genes in a population, which was not specifically addressed in Richard Lenski's ecological models. In order for resistance to spread, transmission is necessary. But we're dealing with phenomena that also affect plasmid persistence, which does in fact mediate the possibility for additional transfer.

With respect to this and in the context of antibiotic cycling, are cycling protocols ever effective in reducing percentage resistance by more than about one order of magnitude? In other words, when we cycle antibiotics so that we see decreases in the prevalence of resistance, are we talking about reductions of just 10–20%?

Lerner: I guess it depends somewhat on the mechanism of resistance, but how fast does the compensation occur in cycling? Suppose you could mandate that on each day of the week you're going use a different antibiotic — would this be effective? Could you pick a short enough time that the compensatory mutations would have not be selected?

Lenski: It's difficult for me to give a simple answer. The problem is if you cycle antibiotics on too short a timescale, while you reduce the opportunity for compensation, you also reduce the amount of time for selection back to sensitivity. I think antibiotic cycling would work best in the situation where you had, for instance, no resistance to penicillin in *Neisseria gonorrhoeae* until the 1970s, and then suddenly you saw the first resistant outbreaks. You would have to quit using penicillin when you saw the first resistant strain, because once it has spread too far you're never going to be able to return to complete susceptibility. But if you can go 'cold turkey' right away, you may buy another 10 years of susceptibility to penicillin before resistance re-appears. This argument presumes that you have an alternative antibiotic that can be used in place of the first one. Otherwise, there's a conflict here between treating the individual patient and protecting the public health by restoring sensitivity.

Cohen: There's a really important point here. Very often when you have the emergence of resistance its persistence and frequency is not only determined by the interaction between antibiotic use and the organisms, but also by the presence of reservoirs for the organism. Thus, if you start cycling it may have little or no impact. We had a nosocomial staphylococcus outbreak in Seattle in the late 1970s in which we observed transmission for over 18 months. Many of the cases of infection could be traced directly or indirectly to one patient who was in an intensive care unit for many months. This patient was a reservoir that effectively colonized various healthcare workers and other patients. The presence of such reservoirs and niches can greatly impact the frequency of resistance in the presence or absence of cycling or antibiotic use.

Witte: In Eastern Germany tetracycline use in animal feeding was suspended in 1983. Within five years the frequency of tetracycline-resistant *E. coli* from urinary tract infections in humans dropped from 46% to 28%. These figures were based on more than 12 000 isolates checked per year. During this time the amount of oxytetracycline used in human medicine didn't change.

Lenski: While it seems impressive that in five years the prevalence of resistance drops from 46% to 28%, if you put the bacteria back under positive antibiotic selection you have probably only bought yourself an extra week! It seems to be much easier to get resistant 'bugs' than to get rid of them.

Huovinen: In a clinical situation it's not very easy to recycle, because there are few options. For example, for group A streptococci there are only four drugs.

Bennish: The model suggests that if cycling of antimicrobials is to be effective, then one should cycle before any resistance arises.

Levy: One can also think of this concept not in terms of the drugs we have now but in terms of lessons to be learned for use of future drugs.

Levin: I want to make a plug for the use of mathematical models for these endeavours. The antibiotic resistance business, as I perceive it, is strong in talk and intuition and weak in hard numbers and formal theory. For example, we would like to know not only that antibiotic-mediated selection will favour the ascent of resistant organisms, but also how long it will take before the frequency of resistance will reach problematic levels. We'd also like to know the rate of descent of resistance genes and plasmids, when the intensity of antibiotic-mediated selection is reduced to specific levels. For well-defined situations, these rates can in fact be calculated by using mathematical models with empirical estimates of their parameters. I see no other way of determining these rates.

Bennish: The other side of the modelling question is that the assumptions in modelling are often not solid enough to convince the users. You can't get someone to change their habits merely by quantifying *your* intuition.

Levin: I'm not suggesting that we should use differential equations to convince patients to follow a particular treatment regime. What I am suggesting is that these equations and models, after appropriate evaluation and parameter estimation, should be employed to develop antibiotic use policy for both individual patients and the community at large. Basing this policy solely on non-quantitative intuitive yak-yak is irresponsible.

Summers: As Bruce is advocating the modelling business, I want to advocate bacterial genetics. The fundamental reservoir of resistance is something that's built into what a lot of us are concerned about: the multiply-resistant plasmid-borne element in which there is genetic linkage. Not only in the models but also in much of the discourse that I've heard here, there's been focus on a single antibiotic resistance gene without regard to what else is going on that linkage group.

Baquero: Cycling is very difficult because there are only a few families of antibiotics, leaving us with few alternatives. We need many new types of antibiotics to counteract the resistance problem from many different families.

Bennish: Chances rarely come twice. We have had more classes of antimicrobial agents available to us in the 1980s than we are likely to have in the foreseeable future.

Cohen: Many of the antibiotic classes that we have are derived from natural sources or modifications thereof, which may make it more likely for resistance to occur. Perhaps we really need more rational antibiotic design based on molecular biology, where we can develop things which don't occur in nature.

Lerner: We're talking about the fact that perhaps we should be cycling agents before the resistance to them arises. If we do get a second effective agent in the future against MRSA in addition to vancomycin, should we be planning ahead to cycle between it and vancomycin?

Lipsitch: Treatment of MRSA patients with vancomycin would probably not be the major selective force in favour of vancomycin-resistant staphylococci in hospitals. Treatment of other infections may be the more important selective force in favour of antibiotic resistance in bacterial species that are transmitted, for the most part, between colonized hosts who are not symptomatic.

Levy: What you're saying is that the selective event is not the vancomycin usage for MRSA.

Lipsitch: It is vancomycin usage against other infections that happens to exert selection on staphylococci that are colonizing the patients asymptomatically.

Levy: If a rare vancomycin-resistant MRSA emerges in a patient and you are using antibiotic B, the organism is eliminated, you are saved. However, if you're using vancomycin for many different conditions and a resistant MRSA emerges, you're in trouble.

Copeland: One of the problems is that if we were to get a new class or new type of antibiotic, then people would want to save it and would therefore be reluctant to use it. One of the difficulties for the pharmaceutical industry is looking for something which ostensibly is not going to be used.

References

Barber M, Dutton AAC, Beard MA, Elmes PC, Williams R 1960 Reversal of antibiotic resistance in hospital staphylococcal infection. Br Med J 1:11–17

Bouma JE, Lenski RE 1988 Evolution of a bacteria/plasmid association. Nature 335:351–352

Cheng J, Baldwin K, Guffanti AA, Krulwich TA 1996 Na^+/H^+ antiport activity conferred by *Bacillus subtilis tetA* (L), a 5' truncation product of *tetA* (L) and mutated plasmid genes upon *Escherichia coli*. Antimicrob Agents Chemother 40:852–857

Condit R, Levin BR 1990 The evolution of plasmids carrying multiple resistance genes: the role of segregation, transposition, and homologous recombination. Am Nat 135:573–596

Crumplin GC 1986 Resistance to DNA gyrase inhibitors. J Med Microbiol 21:R6

Dalhoff A, Doring G 1985 Interference of ciprofloxacin with the expression of pathogenicity factors of *Pseudomonas aeruginosa*. In: Kuhlman J, Dalhoff A, Zeiler HJ (eds) The influence of antibiotics on the host–parasite relationship, vol 2. Springer-Verlag, New York, p 246–255

Lehnherr H, Yarmolinsky MD 1995 Addiction protein Phd of plasmid prophage P1 is a substrate of the CLPXP serine protease of *Escherichia coli*. Proc Natl Acad Sci USA 92:3274–3277

Lenski RE, Simpson SC, Nguyen TT 1994 Genetic analysis of a plasmid-encoded, host-genotype-specific enhancement of bacterial fitness. J Bacteriol 176:3140–3147

Levy SB 1986 Ecology of antibiotic resistance development. In: Levy SB, Novick RP (eds) Antibiotic resistance genes: ecology, transfer and expression. Cold Spring Harbor Press, NY, p 17–29

Levin BR 1980 Conditions for the existence of R plasmids in bacterial populations. In: Mitsuhashi S, Rosival L, Krcmery V (eds) Antibiotic resistance: transposition and other mechanisms. Springer-Verlag, Berlin, p 197–202

Luzatto L, Schlessinger D, Apirion D 1968 *Escherichia coli*: high resistance or dependence on streptomycin produced by the same allele. Science 161:478–479

Nguyen TNM, Phan QG, Duong LP, Bertrand KP, Lenski RE 1989 Effects of carriage and expression of the Tn*10* tetracycline resistance operon on the fitness of *Escherichia coli* K12. Mol Biol Evol 6:213–225

Roberts M, Elwell LP, Falkow S 1977 Molecular characteristics of two β-lactamase-specifying plasmids isolated from *Neisseria gonorrhoeae*. J Bacteriol 131:557–563

Schrag SJ, Perrot V 1996 Reducing antibiotic resistance. Nature 381:120–121

Travisano M, Mongold JA, Bennett AF, Lenski RE 1995 Experimental tests of the roles of adaptation, chance and history in evolution. Science 267:87–90

Turner PE 1995 Associations between bacteria and conjugative plasmids: model systems for testing evolutionary theory. PhD thesis, Michigan State University, East Lansing, MI, USA

Urban C, Go E, Mariano N et al 1993 Effect of sulbactam on infections caused by imipenem-resistant *Acinetobacter calcoaceticus* biotype *anitratus*. J Infect Dis 167:448–451

Zünd P, Lebek J 1980 Generation time-prolonging R plasmids: correlation between increases in the generation time of *Escherichia coli* caused by R plasmids and their molecular size. Plasmid 3:65–69

The evolution of β-lactamases

Karen Bush

Department of Microbial Biochemistry, Astra Research Center Boston, 128 Sidney Street, Cambridge, MA 02139, USA

Abstract. β-lactamases, the enzymes often associated with resistance to β-lactam antibiotics, are found in most bacterial species. Although these enzymes protected bacteria from naturally occurring β-lactams long before the introduction of synthetic antimicrobial agents, the numbers and varieties of β-lactamases have increased dramatically with the introduction of modern penicillins and cephalosporins. Over the past twenty years it has become apparent that families of β-lactamases have been selected as the result of antimicrobial usage. Outbreaks of β-lactam-resistant bacteria can be traced to the introduction of specific classes of β-lactams or to the introduction of a specific agent. Many of the most serious epidemics can be related to transferable β-lactamase genes that are harboured on multidrug-resistant plasmids. The separation of β-lactamases into three major functional groups or four structural classes has been proposed. Stepwise selection of variants within several of these classes has been documented both in the clinical setting and in the laboratory, e.g. the extended-spectrum (TEM and SHV) β-lactamases and the inhibitor-resistant (TEM) β-lactamases. Close relationships among the recently described plasmid-mediated 'cephamycinases' and the common chromosomal cephalosporinases have been identified. Carbapenem-hydrolysing metallo-β-lactamases with broad spectrum hydrolysing activity have become serious concerns as they begin to be described on plasmids. Factors contributing to selection of β-lactam-resistant strains include decreased outer membrane permeability and increased β-lactamase production.

1997 Antibiotic resistance: origins, evolution, selection and spread. Wiley, Chichester (Ciba Foundation Symposium 207) p 152–166

β-lactamases, bacterial enzymes that hydrolyse the amide bond of β-lactam-containing antimicrobial agents, appear to be essential for bacterial survival only when the producing organisms are in the presence of β-lactams. Most bacterial species can synthesize at least one of the more than 200 uniquely described β-lactamases, with a few notable exceptions that include *Streptococcus pneumoniae* and *Helicobacter pylori* (Bush et al 1995, Livermore 1995). Although attempts have been made to assign functions to these enzymes other than β-lactam hydrolysis (Livermore 1995), no convincing evidence has yet been provided to demonstrate other enzymic functions that occur under physiological conditions. High catalytic efficiencies for the hydrolysis of penicillins or cephalosporins, with k_{cat} values as high as $2400\,sec^{-1}$ (Christensen et al 1990) suggest that these enzymes have evolved to perform β-lactam hydrolysis at rates approaching those for diffusion-controlled reactions.

β-lactamase classification

Catalysis of β-lactam hydrolysis occurs with addition of a water molecule across the β-lactam bond, via one of two mechanisms, depending upon the structural type of enzyme. This can happen either by acylating a serine at the active site of a β-lactamase or by using a water molecule coordinated to a zinc-containing active site of a metallo-β-lactamase. β-lactamases have been crudely divided into two structural groups on the basis of this division between metalloenzymes and enzymes that utilize serine at the active site. A slightly more elaborate structural separation scheme based on amino acid sequences of a limited number of β-lactamases was initiated by Ambler (1980), resulting in four currently recognized structural classes: the 'serine β-lactamases' in classes A, C, and D, and the metallo-β-lactamases in class B.

Functional classifications of the β-lactamases have been described by a number of investigators over the past 25 years, including the Richmond & Sykes (1973) classification scheme, and the most comprehensive groupings to date described in 1995 by Bush, Jacoby and Medeiros (Bush et al 1995). Functional groupings are based upon substrate profiles, including the specificity for penicillin or cephalosporin hydrolysis, and upon ability to be inhibited by active site-directed (suicide) inhibitors such as clavulanic acid or by protein modifying agents such as EDTA or p-chloromercuribenzoate. Attempts were made in the 1995 compilation to correlate structural and functional characteristics of 190 β-lactamases deemed to be unique, either in structure or in function. The relationship between the structural and functional groupings is shown in Fig. 1. Molecular class A β-lactamases include the Group 2 functional group of β-lactamases, enzymes with serine at the active site that can be inactivated by clavulanic acid, a representative of the commercially available β-lactamase inhibitors. Group 2 enzymes include many of the most common β-lactamases including the staphylococcal penicillinases and the broad spectrum plasmid-mediated enzymes such as the TEM-1 and SHV-1 enzymes. The class C β-lactamases, or functional group 1 β-lactamases, are enzymes with a larger molecular size than the other monomeric β-lactamases and act functionally as cephalosporinases that are poorly inhibited by clavulanic acid. Class D, or functional group 2d, β-lactamases, enzymes with low sequence homology to other serine β-lactamases, hydrolyse substrates such as oxacillin and cloxacillin. The class B metalloenzymes, or functional group 3 β-lactamases, presently include 15 uniquely described enzymes whose most notable function is to hydrolyse carbapenems (Rasmussen & Bush 1996). These enzymes are inhibited by EDTA but not by the serine-directed inhibitors.

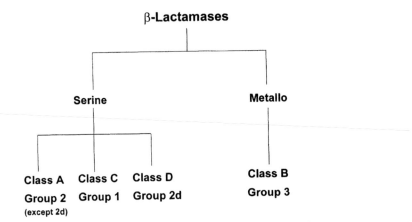

FIG. 1.   Correlation of molecular and functional classification schemes for β-lactamases.

Relationships to penicillin-binding proteins

Most β-lactamases are serine β-lactamases with at least three highly conserved functional and structural elements (Lamotte-Brasseur et al 1994). These elements are conserved as well among the related penicillin-binding proteins (PBPs), bacterial enzymes that catalyse the terminal steps of cell wall synthesis. Relationships among these elements are highlighted in Table 1. Most notable is the active site sequence S-X-X-K which is conserved among all the penicillin interactive proteins that form acyl enzymes with β-lactams. The (S/Y)-X-(N/S/C) sequence involves amino acids that appear to have side chains extending into the active site. The third element, (K/R/H)-(T/S)-G, lies on the opposite wall of the active site. In addition, 3D analyses show very similar shapes for β-lactamases and the D,D-peptidase.

The structural relationship between serine β-lactamases and PBPs is more than coincidental. For a serine β-lactamase, penicillin is frequently an excellent substrate with a low K_m and a high k_{cat} value. But penicillin also functions as an active site acylating agent for PBPs that have a low turnover number (k_{cat}), resulting in PBPs unable to execute their essential role in cell division. It is commonly accepted that penicillin (and, by analogy, other β-lactam-containing antibacterial agents) mimics the natural PBP transpeptidase substrate with its D-Ala-D-Ala terminus (Tipper & Strominger 1965). For most essential PBPs rapid acylation by penicillin at the active site serine is followed by a relatively long-lived acyl complex with a half-life for deacylation that is longer than the doubling time for bacterial growth (Frère et al 1992). As a result bacteria cannot replicate.

Serine β-lactamases may be viewed as PBPs with efficient rates of deacylation for β-lactams. From an evolutionary perspective, PBPs include essential bifunctional enzymes, whereas β-lactamases tend to be 'secondary' smaller molecular weight

TABLE 1 Sequence relationships among penicillin interactive proteins with serine at the active site

Penicillin interactive proteins	Element 1	Element 2	Element 3
Class A β-lactamases	70 S-X-X-K	130 S-D-N S-D-S	234 K-T-G K-S-G R-S-G R-T-G
Class C β-lactamases	64 S-X-X-K	150 Y-A-N	314 K-T-G
Class D β-lactamases	70 S-X-X-K	144 Y-G-N	214 K-T-G
R61 D,D-peptidase	62 S-X-X-K	159 Y-S-N	298 H-T-G
Penicillin-binding proteins	S-X-X-K	S-X-N S-X-C Y-G-N	K-T-G K-S-G

enzymes related to the transpeptidase domain of a PBP. Although PBPs must be functional for bacteria to complete cell division, β-lactamases may have evolved primarily to protect soil bacteria from production of β-lactams by other microorganisms in their environments. Fungi, actinomycetes and bacteria from soil isolates have all been identified as β-lactam-producing organisms (Wells et al 1982). Although many of the β-lactams produced are unstable when purified, it is quite likely that in their natural setting they could be taken up by surrounding bacteria simultaneously with essential nutrients. If soil bacteria produced enzymes with high catalytic activities for β-lactam hydrolysis, the β-lactamase-producing bacteria would have a clear evolutionary advantage over non-β-lactamase-producing organisms.

β-lactamases and β-lactam development

The first modern β-lactamase to be described specifically was an enzyme from *Bacillus* (now, *Escherichia*) *coli*, identified by Abraham & Chain (1940). However, shortly thereafter, the first β-lactamases associated with clinical resistance were penicillinases identified from *Staphylococcus aureus* (Kirby 1944). It is estimated that in the 1940s, when benzylpenicillin was first introduced into clinical use, only 5–8% of the *S. aureus* isolates were penicillinase producers (Kirby 1945); now, 80–90% of the *S. aureus* isolates are penicillin resistant due to plasmid acquisition or because of selection of β-lactamase-producing strains (Kernodle et al 1989). It should be noted that resistance is not due to a single enzyme produced by all *S. aureus* isolates, but to a family of closely related β-lactamases with high specificity for hydrolysis of penicillins and selective, poor, hydrolysis of cephalosporins. Consequently, penicillin, a drug introduced primarily to target Gram-positive bacteria, was made virtually unusable for staphylococcal infections due to the selection of β-lactamase-producing bacteria.

During the late 1950s the 'novel' β-lactams 6-aminopenicillanic acid and cephalosporin C were identified as natural products, serving as the foundations for the subsequent development of semi-synthetic β-lactams capable of withstanding hydrolysis by the staphylococcal β-lactamases. Stable penicillins such as methicillin and oxacillin were developed, as were the 'first generation' cephalosporins such as cephalothin and cefazolin introduced in the early 1960s. The latter cephalosporins with very slow hydrolysis by the *S. aureus* enzymes were also clinically effective against common Gram-negative pathogens including *E. coli* and *Klebsiella pneumoniae*. However, it cannot be coincidental that almost simultaneously broad spectrum β-lactamases and cephalosporinases began to be identified in resistant Gram-negative isolates, as new challenges arose for the β-lactam-containing agents.

Gram-negative bacteria, with a few exceptions, produce chromosomally mediated cephalosporinases, enzymes that can hydrolyse the early cephalosporins at rapid rates. In contrast to the staphylococcal penicillinases, these enzymes have low k_{cat} values for catalysis of penicillin hydrolysis, and generally exhibit relatively low K_m values for penicillins (Galleni & Frère 1988). These enzymes are often present in strains with the potential for induction of high levels of β-lactamases (Sanders & Sanders 1979, Minami et al 1983). Induction, a reversible process, however, became less of a problem with time, as stably derepressed mutants of these organisms were selected, with the capability of producing exceedingly high amounts of cephalosporinase activity. For example, in highly induced or in derepressed mutants of *E. cloacae,* as much as 4% of the soluble protein can be β-lactamase (Bush et al 1985). In addition, derepressed mutants were often found to have decreased permeability through the outer membrane, resulting in slow uptake and subsequent hydrolysis of poor substrates in organisms with elevated β-lactamase levels. As cephalosporins were used more frequently to treat Gram-negative infections, chromosomal cephalosporinases became a more important component of the bacterial armamentarium to attack β-lactams.

By the mid-to-late 1960s concomitant with increased cephalosporin use plasmid-mediated β-lactamases began to be identified in Gram-negative bacteria. Many of these enzymes, including SHV-1 and the ubiquitous TEM-1 or TEM-2 β-lactamases, are broad spectrum enzymes with similar hydrolysis rates for benzylpenicillin and cephaloridine, a 'first generation' cephalosporin (Bush et al 1995). SHV-1 can appear on either the chromosome or on a plasmid, whereas plasmids generally provide the location for the two TEM enzymes that are functionally equivalent and differ by a single amino acid at position 39, distant from the active site. The TEM-1 enzyme, a particularly nasty threat, has been identified in most genera of Gram-negative bacteria. This enzyme became a clinical problem of major proportions when the TEM-encoding gene appeared on a plasmid in *Neisseria gonorrhoeae* (Phillips 1976), thereby rendering a single shot of penicillin ineffective for the treatment of gonorrhea. In a later study, 87.5% of 680 consecutive Enterobacteriaceae isolates produced TEM-1 β-lactamases as identified by isoelectric focusing (Roy et al 1985).

During the mid- to late-1970s the TEM enzymes became the prime target for pharmaceutical discovery programs in the β-lactam arena. Two approaches were attempted: first, identify a potent β-lactamase inhibitor targeting, in particular, the TEM enzyme(s), or, second, develop β-lactam-containing antimicrobial agents stable to enzymic hydrolysis. The first approach resulted in the discovery of the β-lactam-containing clavulanic acid from *Streptomyces clavuligerus* (Brown et al 1976), and the subsequent development of the penicillin-derived sulfone β-lactamase inhibitors sulbactam and tazobactam, all of which were combined with a β-lactamase-labile penicillin in marketable β-lactam combinations. The second approach resulted in the identification of β-lactamase-stable molecules such as the carbapenems from natural isolates, in addition to the selection and development of the stable semi-synthetic 'third generation' cephalosporins cefotaxime, ceftazidime, and cefoperazone, followed by the monobactam aztreonam. The inhibitors were shown to be potent suicide inactivators for the staphylococcal penicillinases and the broad spectrum TEM enzymes (Knowles 1985). The 'β-lactamase stable' molecules were hydrolysed only very slowly, if at all detectably, by all the common β-lactamases described at the time of the development of the expanded spectrum agents (Sykes et al 1982). Enzymologists were forced to purify large quantities of enzyme and use the most sensitive methodology available to measure the very slow rates of hydrolysis observed for many of these compounds (personal observation). It appeared as though the pharmaceutical industry had accomplished their mission to circumvent the action of β-lactamases. However, these well-calculated events had their own consequences.

β-lactamase variants

Following the introduction of the expanded spectrum cephalosporins such as cefotaxime in 1981 and ceftazidime in 1985 (US approval dates), many hospitals switched to these as first line therapy. Soon thereafter in Western Europe, Gram-negative bacteria were documented to carry transferable resistance to these agents, with the first reports of an 'extended-spectrum β-lactamase,' or, ESBL, identified from Germany in 1983 (Knothe et al 1983) and in France shortly afterward (Sirot et al 1987). Major outbreaks were recorded in France beginning in 1984 (Sirot et al 1991) and in the United States beginning in 1988 (Meyer et al 1993). In the latter outbreak 155 patients were infected with ceftazidime- and aztreonam-resistant *K. pneumoniae* isolates over a two year period. Cefotaxime and ceftazidime, used heavily in the affected hospitals, were subsequently shown to select for variants of the TEM and SHV β-lactamases. These mutant enzymes, conferring resistant phenotypes or causing elevated minimum inhibitory concentrations (MICs) to be observed in the producing

TABLE 2   Hydrolysis of selected substrates by extended-spectrum β-lactamases

Enzyme	Amino acid substitution(s)[a]	Relative hydrolysis rate			
		Benzylpenicillin	Cephaloridine	Cefotaxime	Ceftazidime
TEM-1		100	140	0.07	0.01
TEM-2	Q39K	100	120	0.08	<0.01
TEM-3	Q39K, E104K, G238S	100	120	170	8.3
TEM-5	R164S, A237T, E240K	100	300	29	100
TEM-7	Q39K, R164S	100	120	1.9	1.7
TEM-10	R164S, E240K	100	77	1.6	68
TEM-12	R164S	100	57	2.4	3.8
TEM-20	G328S	100	150	250	<1
TEM-26	E104K, R164S	100	120	7.5	170
SHV-1		100	48	0.18	0.02
SHV-2	G238S	100	130	19	0.51
SHV-4	R205L, G238S, E240K	100	5.6	1.1	0.65
SHV-7	I8F, R43S, G238S, E240K	100	91	30	13

[a]Compared with TEM-1 for the TEM-derived enzymes and SHV-1 for the SHV-derived enzymes. Data adapted from Bush et al (1995) and Knox (1995).

organisms, contained one to four amino acid changes that resulted from point mutations in the nucleotide sequences in the parent genes (Knox 1995).

At the present time five SHV variants have been identified, SHV-2 to SHV-5 and SHV-7 (Bradford et al 1995). The activities of these enzymes vary from (1) moderate to weak hydrolysis of cefotaxime and low hydrolysis of ceftazidime for SHV-2, to (2) moderate hydrolysis of both cephalosporins by SHV-7 (Table 2). In comparison, many more TEM variants associated with hydrolysis of the expanded spectrum β-lactam-containing agents have been identified: a minimum of 22 unique TEM sequences based on TEM-1 have one to four amino acid changes (TEM-3 to TEM-29 and TEM-42). The alignment of related SHV and TEM variants is shown in Fig. 2. Only the G238S and the E240K substitutions occur in both the TEM- and SHV-derived variants. The enzymic activity of the TEM-derived ESBLs can vary widely, with some enzymes preferring to hydrolyse cefotaxime, e.g. TEM-3 and TEM-20 with the G238S substitution, and other ESBLs showing preference for hydrolysis of ceftazidime, e.g. TEM-10 and TEM-26. TEM-derived enzymes that contain only a single amino acid change at position 164, compared to either the TEM-1 or TEM-2 β-lactamases, have elevated hydrolysis of these two expanded spectrum cephalosporins compared to the parent, but need a second mutation to achieve high levels of

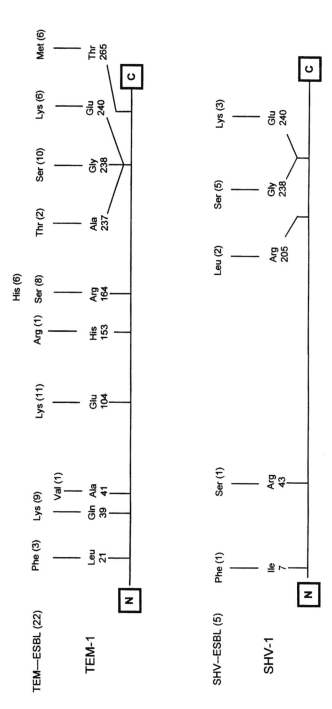

FIG. 2. Amino acid substitutions in 22 extended-spectrum β-lactamases (ESBLs) derived from the TEM-1 β-lactamase and in five ESBLs derived from the SHV-1 β-lactamase. Numbers in parentheses represent the number of enzymes with the specified substitutions.

hydrolysis (Table 2). It should be noted that all the ESBLs have retained the ability to be inhibited by the commercially available active site inhibitors.

Following the approval of the amoxicillin/clavulanic acid combination in the United States in 1984 and the later approval of ampicillin/sulbactam in 1986, the use of a β-lactamase inhibitor with a penicillin appeared to be an excellent strategy to delay resistance development. In fact, resistance to the inhibitors has taken a longer time to develop than resistance to a single β-lactam-containing agent, with smaller populations of organisms affected. To date, variant TEM β-lactamases with decreased affinity for the inhibitors have been confined primarily to Western Europe, e.g. France and Spain with a few isolates from the United Kingdom (Henquell et al 1995, Stapleton et al 1995). These enzymes are derived from the TEM-1 β-lactamase with only one to three amino acid changes, none of which has yet been published as occurring in an ESBL. Inhibitor resistance appears to be most closely correlated with amino acid changes at Met69, adjacent to the active site serine, or at Arg244. In laboratory studies, in fact, a TEM enzyme with mutations associated with both ESBL activity, R164S, and inhibitor resistance, R244S, is capable of hydrolysing ceftazidime but is fully susceptible to inhibition by clavulanic acid (Imitiaz et al 1994). Therefore, selection of ESBLs with inhibitor-resistant characteristics may be difficult.

Cephamycins, 3-methoxycephalosporins initially identified from a soil isolate, are β-lactams with good stability to hydrolysis by all the TEM β-lactamases. Semisynthetic derivatives such as cefoxitin were developed to withstand β-lactamase-mediated resistance. Following clinical use, however, the result was to select for organisms that produced cephalosporinases capable of slowly hydrolysing the cephamycins. In addition, cefoxitin was shown to be a potent inducer of the chromosomal cephalosporinases in Enterobacteriaceae (Minami et al 1983), resulting in very high β-lactamase levels. Recently, close relatives of genes encoding these enzymes have been identified on high copy number plasmids resulting in cephalosporinases somewhat more proficient in cephamycin hydrolysis (Bauernfeind et al 1990, Leiza et al 1994).

Imipenem, approved for US clinical use in 1985, is one of the most potent single antimicrobial agents available for therapy. This carbapenem is derived from thienamycin, a natural product isolated from an actinomycete (Kahan et al 1979). It should be no surprise, therefore, that β-lactamases capable of hydrolysing carbapenems were in existence long before the use of imipenem. However, it is only with more widespread clinical use of this agent that an increasing variety of carbapenem-hydrolysing enzymes are being identified, including plasmid-mediated varieties from Japan (Rasmussen & Bush 1996). Selected serine β-lactamases and all metallo-β-lactamases are capable of utilizing carbapenems as substrates, but the specific substrate and inhibitor profiles vary considerably. Among the metalloenzymes at least three different functional groups have been proposed, with three different molecular divisions (Rasmussen & Bush 1996). The metalloenzymes are all refractory to inhibition by the commercially available inhibitors. Substrate profiles vary from the group of metallo-β-lactamases that hydrolyse every known class of β-lactams — except monobactams — to the group of enzymes that hydrolyse only carbapenems well but not cephalosporins or penicillins. Only a small group of carbapenem-hydrolysing enzymes have been identified with serine at the active site: five isolates producing three distinct enzymes have been characterized, representing one of the smallest functional and structural groups of β-lactamases (Bush et al 1995). Again, it is noteworthy that two of these three enzymes appeared in isolates before imipenem was used commercially.

Future concerns

Some have predicted that the era of β-lactams is over: no new β-lactam-containing agent will be able to circumvent the β-lactamases that can be elaborated by ingenious bacteria. In addition to the extensive variety of substrate profiles exhibited by more than 200 β-lactamases, genes encoding the enzymes have been hopping out of chromosomes onto plasmids and then back onto the chromosome, resulting in virtually unrestrained transferability of many enzymes. However, β-lactams have proven to be safe, efficacious, inexpensive, broad spectrum antibacterial agents with a high 'comfort level' associated with their use. In spite of the versatility of the enzymes capable of hydrolysing the spectrum of β-lactams, β-lactamase production is still not universal. As shown by the length of time required for resistance to develop to the inhibitor combinations, perhaps the judicious use of β-lactam combinations will decelerate the rate at which new β-lactamases are selected. However, one can, with certainty, predict that bacteria will eventually circumvent any novel antimicrobial agent introduced. Perhaps our most optimistic hope is to try to delay the development of novel β-lactamases in epidemic proportions.

Acknowledgements

This paper evolved as a result of many spirited, and thoughtful, discussions over the past twenty years with friends and colleagues, including particularly Richard Sykes, Antone Medeiros, George Jacoby, Christine Sanders, David Livermore and Fernando Baquero.

References

Abraham EP, Chain E 1940 An enzyme from bacteria able to destroy penicillin. Nature 146:837
Ambler RP 1980 The structure of β-lactamases. Philos Trans R Soc Lond B Biol Sci 289:321–331
Bauernfeind A, Schweighart S, Dornbusch K, Giamarellou H 1990 A transferable cephamycinase in *Klebsiella pneumoniae*. In: Program and abstracts of the 30th Interscience Conference on Antimicrobial Agents and Chemotherapy, Oct 21–24, Atlanta, GA. American Society for Microbiology, Abstr 190
Bradford PA, Urban C, Jaiswal A et al 1995 SHV-7, a novel cefotaxime hydrolysing β-lactamase, identified in *Escherichia coli* isolates from hospitalized nursing home patients. Antimicrob Agents Chemother 39:899–905

Brown AG, Butterworth D, Cole M et al 1976 Naturally occurring β-lactamase inhibitors with antibacterial activity. J Antibiot 29:668–669

Bush K, Tanaka SK, Bonner DP, Sykes RB 1985 Resistance caused by decreased penetration of β-lactam antibiotics into *Enterobacter cloacae*. Antimicrob Agents Chemother 27:555–560

Bush K, Jacoby GA, Medeiros AA 1995 A functional classification scheme for β-lactamases and its correlation with molecular structure. Antimicrob Agents Chemother 39:1211–1233

Christensen H, Martin MT, Waley SG 1990 β-lactamases as fully efficient enzymes. Determination of all the rate constants in the acyl-enzyme mechanism. Biochem J 266:853–861

Frère J-M, Nguyen-Disteche M, Coyette J, Joris B 1992 Mode of action: interaction with the penicillin binding proteins. In: Page MI The chemistry of β-lactams. Chapman & Hall, New York, p 148–197

Galleni M, Frère J-M 1988 A survey of the kinetic parameters of class C β-lactamases. Penicillins. Biochem J 255:119–122

Henquell C, Chanal C, Sirot D, Labia R, Sirot J 1995 Molecular characterization of nine different types of mutants among 107 inhibitor-resistant TEM β-lactamases from clinical isolates of *Escherichia coli*. Antimicrob Agents Chemother 39:427–430

Imitiaz U, Manavathu EK, Mobasherey S, Lerner SA 1994 Reversal of clavulanate resistance conferred by a Ser-244 mutant of TEM-1 β-lactamase as a result of a second mutation (Arg to Ser at position 164) that enhances activity against ceftazidime. Antimicrob Agents Chemother 38:1134–1139

Kahan JS, Kahan FM, Goegelman R et al 1979 Thienamycin, a new β-lactam antibiotic. I. Discovery, taxonomy, isolation and physical properties. J Antibiotics 32:1–12

Kernodle DS, Stratton CW, McMurray LW, Chipley JR, McGraw PA 1989 Differentiation of β-lactamase variants of *Staphylococcus aureus* by substrate hydrolysis profiles. J Infect Dis 159:103–108

Kirby WMM 1944 Extraction of a highly potent penicillin inactivator from penicillin resistant staphylococci. Science 99:452–453

Kirby WMM 1945 Bacteriostatic and lytic actions of penicillin on sensitive and resistant staphylococci. J Clin Invest 24:165–169

Knothe H, Shah P, Krcmery V, Antal M, Mitsuhashi S 1983 Transferable resistance to cefotaxime, cefoxitin, cefamandole and cefuroxime in clinical isolates of *Klebsiella pneumoniae* and *Serratia marcescens*. Infection 11:315–317

Knowles JR 1985 Penicillin resistance: the chemistry of β-lactamase inhibition. Acc Chem Res 18:97–104

Knox JR 1995 Extended-spectrum and inhibitor-resistant TEM-type β-lactamases: mutations, specificity and three-dimensional structure. Antimicrob Agents Chemother 39:2593–2601

Lamotte-Brasseur J, Knox J, Kelly JA et al 1994 The structures and catalytic mechanisms of active-site serine β-lactamases. In: Tombs MP (ed) Biotechnology and genetic engineering reviews, vol 12. Intercept, Andover, p 189–230

Leiza MG, Perez-Diaz JC, Ayala J et al 1994 Gene sequence and biochemical characterization of FOX-1 from *Klebsiella pneumoniae*, a new AmpC-type plasmid-mediated β-lactamase with two molecular variants. Antimicrob Agents Chemother 38:2150–2157

Livermore D 1995 β-Lactamases in laboratory and clinical resistance. Clin Microbiol Rev 8:557–584

Meyer KS, Urban C, Eagan JA, Berger BJ, Rahal JJ 1993 Nosocomial outbreak of *Klebsiella* infection resistant to late-generation cephalosporins. Ann Intern Med 119:353–358

Minami S, Matsubara N, Yotsuji A et al 1983 Induction of cephalosporinase production by various penicillins in Enterobacteriaceae. J Antibiot 36:1387–1395

Phillips I 1976 β-lactamase producing, penicillin-resistant gonococcus. Lancet II:656–657

Rasmussen BA, Bush K 1996 Carbapenem-hydrolyzing β-lactamases. Antimicrob Agents Chemother 40: 223–231

Richmond MH, Sykes RB 1973 The β-lactamases of gram-negative bacteria and their possible physiological role. In: Rose AH, Tempest DW (eds) Advances in microbial physiology, vol 9. Academic Press, New York, p 31–88

Roy C, Segura C, Tirado M et al 1985 Frequency of plasmid-determined β-lactamases in 680 consecutively isolated strains of *Enterobacteriaceae*. Eur J Clin Microbiol 4:146–147

Sanders CC, Sanders WE 1979 Emergence of resistance to cefamandole: possible role of cefoxitin-inducible β-lactamases. Antimicrob Agents Chemother 15:792–797

Sirot D, Sirot J, Labia R et al 1987 Transferable resistance to third-generation cephalosporins in clinical isolates of *Klebsiella pneumoniae*: identification of CTX-1, a novel β-lactamase. J Antimicrob Chemother 20:323–334

Sirot D, DeChamps C, Chanal C et al 1991 Translocation of antibiotic resistance determinants including an extended-spectrum β-lactamase between conjugative plasmids of *Klebsiella pneumoniae* and *Escherichia coli*. Antimicrob Agents Chemother 35:1576–1581

Stapleton P, Wu P-J, King A, Shannon K, French G, Phillips I 1995 Incidence and mechanisms of resistance to the combination of amoxicillin and clavulanic acid in *Escherichia coli*. Antimicrob Agents Chemother 39:2478–2483

Sykes RB, Bonner DP, Bush K, Georgopapadakou NH 1982 Azthreonam (SQ 26,776), a synthetic monobactam specifically active against aerobic gram-negative bacteria. Antimicrob Agents Chemother 21:85–92

Tipper DJ, Strominger JL 1965 Mechanism of action of penicillins: a proposal based on their structural similarity to acyl-D-alanyl-D-alanine. Proc Natl Acad Sci USA 54:1133–1141

Wells JS, Hunter JC, Astle GL et al 1982 Distribution of β-lactam and β-lactone producing bacteria in nature. J Antibiotics 35:814–821

DISCUSSION

Lerner: The most common replacements in the ESBLs from TEM are serine and histidine for arginine at position 164. We looked at all the other mutations at 164 and found that kinetically and microbiologically a mutant enzyme with asparagine at that site confers the highest resistance, and we wondered why this mutation hadn't been found in nature. It turns out that replacement by asparagine requires two mutations from the arginine codon, whereas the serine and histidine mutant enzymes, which are almost as good as the mutant with asparagine, require only one nucleotide change.

Davies: If β-lactamases are produced by soil microbes to protect themselves against the action of β-lactam antibiotics in soil, has anyone found β-lactam antibiotics in soil?

Bush: Yes; monobactams are found free in soil. When organisms were grown for monobactam production, cells grew to the point where they were in stationary phase, where they were beginning to secrete metabolites. The basis for the Squibb identification of monobactams was secretion of the β-lactam into the culture medium. The general consensus is that they would also be secreted into a natural (soil) environment.

Davies: I know that the producing organisms are found in the soil — I want to know whether there is free β-lactam antibiotic in the soil.

Bush: That I don't know, but there is free antibiotic released into culture media.

Huovinen: If I remember correctly, TEM-1 was found in three places simultaneously in the early 1960s. What is the origin of this gene?

Bush: I've had this discussion with several β-lactamase experts. One hypothesis described by Roger Labia's group (Barthélémy et al 1988) begins with selected strains of *Klebsiella pneumoniae* that produce a chromosomal β-lactamase, such as the LEN-1 enzyme. This enzyme is 88% homologous to the SHV-1 β-lactamase, an enzyme that can be encoded either on the chromosome of some *Klebsiella* strains, or on plasmids. The SHV-1 enzyme is 68% homologous to the plasmid-mediated TEM-1. Therefore, it is possible that the TEM-1 enzyme derived from a chromosomal *Klebsiella* enzyme going through SHV-1 as an intermediate.

Hall: Are you arguing that SHV was originally a chromosomal *Klebsiella* gene?

Bush: Yes.

Hall: I would like to see some corroborating evidence for that!

Bush: It's frequently found in the chromosome of *Klebsiella pneumoniae* isolates.

Hall: Anything on a transposon can be frequently found in a bacterial chromosome. I'm not saying it is not chromosomal, but there are ways of asking whether it is, such as whether it looks similar to other *Klebsiella* genes.

TEM-1, TEM-2 and TEM-3 are all found on the same transposon. They are from different plasmids all isolated at similar times from different countries. Doesn't that suggest that the TEMs already occurred world-wide at the time they first emerged in clinical isolates?

Baquero: Even within TEM-1 there may be different evolutionary lineages: TEM-1A and 1B differ by three nucleotides, and these derive from transposons Tn*3* and Tn*2*, respectively.

Hall: That only supports my argument that they had been around for a long time before they were isolated. They must have been separated long enough to accumulate mutational differences. If TEM and SHV are 80% similar they are 20% different, and this is the magnitude of the difference between *E. coli* and *Salmonella*. So if you are going to argue that SHV was originally a *Klebsiella* gene that somehow got into Tn*3* and there has been this divergence, then you're arguing that this happened millions of years ago.

Bush: It could have occurred.

Hall: I'm simply making the statement that you're talking about a long evolutionary distance at that kind of separation, so the emergence of these different genes is likely to have occurred long before the introduction of antibiotics to clinical therapy.

Lenski: Might you get some indication of the ancestry from the pattern of codon usage? From this you might also get some idea of whether the transposon goes back very deep in several different lineages as opposed to having spread horizontally very recently. There tends to be a convergence in the pattern of codon use by which you can roughly date the movement of genes into a particular species or group.

Hall: For TEM, which is what we are currently discussing, you are talking about only very few base changes.

Lenski: Could you test the hypothesis that SHV had a *Klebsiella* ancestry by looking at codon usage?

Hall: Yes, but nobody has done it so far as I know.

Davies: TEM-2 has been shown to have a stronger promoter than TEM-1. How often are up-promoter mutations unrelated to TEM-2 found on plasmids which encode β-lactamases?

Bush: Hyperproduction of TEM-1 will result in resistance to the β-lactamase inhibitors, a frequent cause for clinical resistance to penicillin–inhibitor combinations.

Lerner: Have the promoters been looked at?

Bush: There are studies showing that mutations in the Pribnow box are related to up-promotion of β-lactamases (Fournier et al 1995).

Levy: Here we are witnessing evolution. Are we seeing mutation in action, or are we seeing the recruitment of genes that have been out there in low numbers and are being brought up to prominence?

Summers: What about the genetic vehicles involved in this? Is there a correlation of any kind that some loci tend to be involved with certain kinds of genetic vehicles as opposed to other kinds?

Bush: In the Chicago outbreak of TEM-10 β-lactamases we found both Tn*2* and Tn*3* origins for the TEM-1 sequences (Rasmussen et al 1993).

Hall: Tn*2* and Tn*3* are very closely related transposons; their overall structure is identical and there are a limited number of base changes, which permits you to distinguish them. Both TEM sequences ought to have the capacity to mutate; so it is not very surprising that mutants arising from both are seen.

Summers: How often is it the case that the TEMs are part of an integron type thing? It is presumably not common.

Hall: They are usually part of Tn*3*/Tn*1*/Tn*2*/Tn α, not an integron, but these transposons (i.e. Tn*3* etc.) and integrons frequently co-ride on the same plasmids.

Summers: If the TEMs are riding on something like that, what about the other classes of β-lactamases?

Hall: Other β-lactamases (mostly class D) are encoded in cassettes and found in integrons.

Levy: Have we established that the evolution occurs within the transposon or something looking like the transposon?

Bush: For the TEMs, yes.

Levy: Why are the broad-spectrum TEM β-lactamase genes always found associated with large plasmids bearing multidrug resistance, particularly gentamicin resistance? Some of these TEMs also appear to have preferences for certain organisms. Can we link the potential for mutation to the other genes on the plasmid? Do we know anything about where the mutated genes might have been initially maintained or selected?

Bush: In Clermont-Ferrand, France, the first major outbreak of extended-spectrum β-lactamases was reported. This incidence was correlated with increased amikacin resistance due to the production of AAC6′, during a time in which amikacin use increased. Both the aminoglycoside and β-lactam resistances appeared on the same plasmid, causing the initial speculation that amikacin might be serving as the selecting agent.

Sköld: I would like to ask about the alternative origin of β-lactamases. Aren't there data to show that *ampC* is involved with the turnover of murein in *E. coli?* Mutation of one of the regulatory genes, *ampD*, causes changes in the murein composition. Would you accept this as a lead for an origin of β-lactamases among murein-synthesizing enzymes?

Bush: There is very strong evidence that the regulation of *ampC* β-lactamase is related to cell wall recycling, but the β-lactamase itself isn't. Some investigators are trying to see if there may be another natural β-lactamase substrate. But if you have a β-lactamase substrate that is being turned over 2000 times per second such as benzylpenicillin this suggests that the enzyme has evolved almost to the stage of diffusion-controlled reactions.

Baquero: Bishop & Weiner (1993) studied the deletion of the *ampC* gene in an *E. coli* assay. They showed that in the absence of this gene growth was reduced, particularly at the end of the exponential phase. They suggested that AmpC is acting as a murein hydrolase in this particular strain.

Levy: Does everyone agree with Karen that β-lactamases evolved from PBPs?

Spratt: Yes. Their 3D structures are clearly homologous. The evidence is very convincing.

Summers: I want to raise a note of caution about making too many extrapolations about the evolution of promiscuous plasmid-carried genes. For one thing, every time those genes move to a new genus or species they're are up against the additional selection of restriction enzymes, which operate in prokaryotes all over the place. It is not something evolutionists in the eukaryotic business have to worry about. The other point that is dangerous to overlook is that plasmid-carried genes have evolved to be expressible in many different host backgrounds. Making up phylogenies on the basis of codon utilization might get you some pretty funny answers. If you just take the Tn*21* mercury resistance system I work on, codon utilization is very atypical for *E. coli* even though Tn*21* is often found there. Even within *E. coli*, rare codons are often used to control the expression of genes. Half the genes in the *mer* locus have rare codons in abundance.

References

Barthélémy M, Perduzzi J, Labia R 1988 Complete amino acid sequence of p453-plasmid-mediated PIT-2 β-lactamase (SHV-1). Biochem J 251:73–79

Bishop RE, Weiner JH 1993 Complementation of growth defect in an *ampC* deletion mutant of Escherichia coli. FEMS Microbiol Lett 114:349–354

Fournier B, Lu CY, LaGrange PH, Krishnamoorthy R, Philippon A 1995 Point mutation in the Pribnow box, the molecular basis of β-lactamase overproduction in *Klebsiella oxytoca*. Antimicrob Agents Chemother 39:1365–1368

Rasmussen BA, Bradford PA, Quinn JP, Wiener J, Weinstein RA, Bush K 1993 Genetically diverse ceftazidime resistant isolates from a single center: biochemical and genetic characterization of TEM-10 β-lactamases encoded by different nucleotide sequences. Antimicrob Agents Chemother 37:1989–1992

Molecular evolution of multiply-antibiotic-resistant staphylococci

Ronald A. Skurray and Neville Firth

School of Biological Sciences, Macleay Building A12, University of Sydney, NSW 2006, Australia

Abstract. Methicillin-resistant *Staphylococcus aureus* (MRSA) is an intractable nosocomial pathogen. The chemotherapeutic intransigence of this organism stems from its predilection to antimicrobial resistance as a consequential response to selective pressures prevailing in the clinical environment. MRSA isolates are frequently resistant to all practicable antimicrobials except the glycopeptide, vancomycin. Although antimicrobial resistance sometimes arises via chromosomal mutation, the emergence of multiply-antibiotic-resistant staphylococci is primarily due to the acquisition of pre-existent resistance genes; such determinants can be encoded chromosomally or by plasmids and are often associated with transposons or insertion sequences. Clinical staphylococci commonly carry one or more plasmids, ranging from small replicons that are phenotypically cryptic or contain only a single resistance gene, to larger episomes that possess several such determinants and sometimes additionally encode systems that mediate their own conjugative transmission and the mobilization of other plasmids. The detection of closely related plasmids, elements and/or genes in other hosts, including coagulase-negative staphylococci and enterococci, attests to interspecific and intergeneric genetic exchange facilitated by mobile genetic elements and DNA transfer mechanisms. The extended genetic reservoir accessible to staphylococci afforded by such horizontal gene flux is fundamental to the acquisition, maintenance and dissemination of staphylococcal antimicrobial resistance in general, and multiresistance in particular.

1997 Antibiotic resistance: origins, evolution, selection and spread. Wiley, Chichester (Ciba Foundation Symposium 207) p 167–191

Staphylococci are important aetiological agents of nosocomial infections worldwide. The clinical significance of *Staphylococcus aureus* and coagulase-negative staphylococci (CNS) is primarily a consequence of the resistance typically exhibited by these organisms to the majority of commonly used antimicrobials. Whereas resistance to some agents has arisen via chromosomal mutation (e.g. fusidic acid, rifampicin and streptomycin), in most cases resistance in staphylococci can be attributed to the acquisition of 'pre-evolved' determinants. A selection of the impressive array of antimicrobial resistances now evident in staphylococcal isolates is presented in Table 1. For a recent review of antibiotic resistance in staphylococci, see Paulsen et al (1996).

TABLE 1 Staphylococcal antimicrobial resistance determinants[a]

Determinant	Resistance(s)[b]	Mechanism[c]	Location(s)[d]
aacA–aphD	Gm Tm Km	Modification	p, c, t
aadD	Nm Km	Modification	p
aadE	Sm	Modification	p, c, t
aphA	Nm Km	Modification	p, c, t
arsB/arsC	Arsenite/arsenate	Active export	p, c
blaZ	Penicillin	Inactivation	p, c, t
ble	Bleomycin	Sequestration	c
cadA	Cadmium/zinc	Active export	p
cadB	Cadmium/zinc	Sequestration (?)	p, c
cat	Chloramphenicol	Inactivation	p
dfrA	Trimethoprim	Bypass	p, t?
ermA	MLS	Target alteration	c, t
ermB	MLS	Target alteration	p, t
ermC	MLS	Target alteration	p
grlA	Fluoroquinolones	Target alteration	c
gyrA/B	Fluoroquinolones	Target alteration	c
linA	Lincomycin	Modification	p
mecA	Methicillin	Altered PBP-2′	c, t?
merA/merB	Hg/organomercurials	Detoxification	p, c, t?
msrA	MS	Active export	p
mupA	Mupirocin	Target alteration	p, c
qacA	Organic cations	Active export	p
qacB	Organic cations	Active export	p
smr	Organic cations	Active export	p
rif	Rifampicin	Target alteration	c
spc	Spectinomycin	Modification	c, t
str	Streptomycin	Modification	p
sulA	Sulfonamides	Bypass	c
tetA(K)	Tetracycline	Active export	p
vat	SgA	Modification	p, c
vatB	SgA	Modification	p
vga	SgA	Active export (?)	p
vgb	SgB	Modification	p

[a]Refer to Paulsen et al (1996) for a comprehensive compilation of determinants.
[b]Abbreviations are: Gm, gentamicin; Hg, mercury; Km, kanamycin; MLS, macrolides, lincosamides and streptogramin type B antibiotics; MS, macrolides and streptogramin type B antibiotics; Nm, neomycin; SgA, streptogramin type A compounds; SgB, streptogramin type B compounds; Sm, streptomycin; Sp, spectinomycin; Tm, tobramycin.
[c]In those cases marked with (?), the mechanism of resistance has only been proposed, not experimentally determined.
[d]Abbreviations for gene locations: p, plasmid; c, chromosome; t, transposon; ?, putative.

Resistance genes can be located chromosomally or on the multiple plasmids commonly present in clinical strains, and are frequently located on transposons (Tn) or associated with insertion sequences (IS)(Lyon & Skurray 1987, Paulsen et al 1996). Plasmids, transposable genetic elements and gene transfer mechanisms are presumed to represent the primary vehicles mediating the acquisition and dissemination of antimicrobial resistance in staphylococci. Gene transfer mechanisms in staphylococci include plasmid-mediated conjugation, mixed culture transfer and transduction.

Three main groups of staphylococcal plasmids have been identified; viz., small, multiresistance and conjugative (Novick 1989, Paulsen et al 1996). Genetic and physical maps of representative staphylococcal plasmids are presented in Fig. 1, and selected plasmids are listed in Table 2. The small (1–10 kb) staphylococcal plasmids (class I) characterized to date utilize the rolling circle mode of replication via a ssDNA intermediate and are therefore known as rolling circle (RC) or ssDNA plasmids. These plasmids are multicopy (15–60 copies/cell) and are usually phenotypically cryptic or carry only a single resistance gene. Plasmids of this class often share highly similar DNA segments, such that individual plasmids appear to be mosaic structures consisting of discrete cassettes encoding replication (*rep*), resistance, and sometimes recombination (*pre*) and/or mobilization (*mob*) functions (Novick 1989). The replication strategy of class I plasmids is thought to promote horizontal exchange of these segments. In contrast to the RC plasmids, we have recently identified a distinct group of small plasmids that appear to utilize an iteron-regulated theta mode replicon; these plasmids are termed the pSK639 family after the prototype plasmid, pSK639 (Fig. 1), isolated from a clinical *S. epidermidis* isolate. pSK639 encodes trimethoprim resistance (Tp[r]) and is mobilizable; other members of this family additionally encode a second resistance determinant (S. Apisiridej, A. Leelaporn, C. D. Scaramuzzi, N. Firth and R. A. Skurray, unpublished results, Leelaporn et al 1996).

Class II multiresistance plasmids are typically 15–40 kb in size and are maintained at approximately 4–6 copies/cell. The β-lactamase (Shalita et al 1980) and pSK1 (Lyon & Skurray 1987) families are the most thoroughly characterized types of class II plasmids. These plasmids typically encode multiple antimicrobial resistance genes, often located on one or more transposon-like structures and/or associated with IS elements.

Class III plasmids are also large (30–60 kb) and normally possess a number of resistance determinants but are distinguished by the ability to promote their own conjugative transfer. Conjugative plasmids can also sometimes facilitate the mobilization of other non-conjugative plasmids, such as some class I plasmids (e.g., pC221). A family of structurally related episomes, such as pSK41, pGO1 and pJE1, are the only conjugative plasmids to be studied in any detail (Fig. 1) (Evans & Dyke 1988, Firth et al 1993, Morton et al 1993). Transposable elements are also a common feature of conjugative plasmids. Several conjugative plasmids that are seemingly distinct from the pSK41 family have been detected, but await detailed examination.

A number of transposons and insertion sequences have been identified in staphylococci, often associated in some way with antimicrobial resistance genes

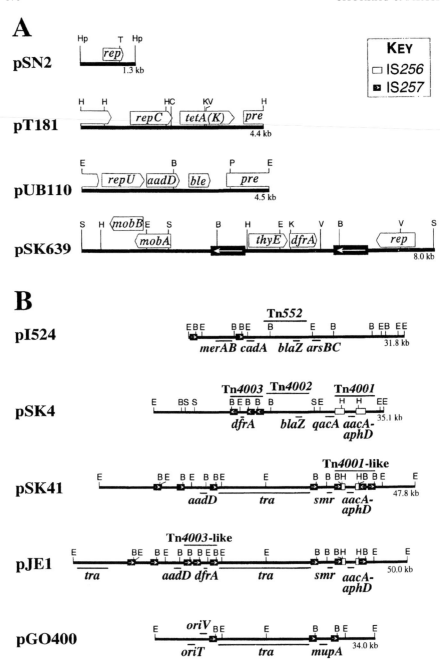

(Table 3) (Murphy 1988, Paulsen et al 1996). Whereas the transposition of some of these has been formally demonstrated (e.g. Tn*4001* and Tn*552*), the mobility of others, such as the IS*257*-associated composite structures (e.g. Tn*4003* and Tn*4291*) are presumed to be mobile based on the detection of typical features; viz., flanking target duplications, terminal inverted repeats, presence of an open reading frame (ORF) encoding a transposase homologue, and/or identification in varied genetic contexts.

IS*257*-mediated co-integrative capture of resistance determinants

The 0.79 kb insertion sequence, IS*257* (Rouch & Skurray 1989), has been found in association with a number of antimicrobial resistance determinants located both on plasmids or the chromosome of staphylococci (Table 4), and copies also flank a transfer-associated region (*tra*) of conjugative plasmids (Figs 1 and 2)(Byrne et al 1990a,b, Stewart et al 1994). IS*257* therefore appears to have played a particularly significant role in the development of resistance in this group of organisms. Studies, by us and others, of IS*257* in various genetic contexts, have revealed several activities attributable to this element, and highlighted potentially related properties that appear to explain the prevalence and organization of IS*257* copies on various replicons. Such investigations represent an enlightening case-study in the context of the development of staphylococcal antimicrobial resistance, particularly multiresistance; the insights provided and the evolutionary implications arising from them form the major focus of this paper.

Although detected on all classes of plasmids, the prevalence of IS*257* is most striking on conjugative plasmids of the pSK41 family (Figs 1 and 2A) and to a lesser extent the chromosome of some *S. aureus* strains (Fig. 2B). In several instances, such as the aminoglycoside resistance determinant *aadD* on pSK41, antibiotic resistance genes flanked by IS*257* have been found to correspond to integrated copies of small plasmids (pUB110 in the case of *aadD* on pSK41; Fig. 2A; Table 5)(Byrne et al 1991, Dubin et al 1991, Gillespie et al 1986). The presence of directly repeated copies of IS*257* flanking such structures implicates this element in the event(s) responsible for co-integration. Furthermore, 8 bp repeat sequences within the co-integrated plasmid in some cases (Fig. 2), adjacent to the flanking IS*257* elements, probably represent target duplications suggestive of transposition of this element as a stage in co-

---

FIG. 1. (*opposite*) Representative staphylococcal plasmids. Physical and genetic maps of representative small (A) and multiresistance (B) plasmids are shown. The sizes of the respective plasmids are indicated on the right. The positions and extents of particular transposons are indicated. The orientation of IS*257* is denoted by an arrow in the solid box. Arrowed boxes above the restriction maps indicate the extents and directions of genes in A, and lines beneath the restriction maps show the extents of the indicated genes/regions in B. See Tables 1, 2 and 3 and text for details of genes, plasmid classifications and transposable elements. Selected restriction sites shown are: B, *Bgl*II; C, *Cla*I; E, *Eco*RI; H, *Hin*dIII; Hp, *Hpa*II; K, *Kpn*I; P, *Pvu*II; S, *Sal*I; T, *Taq*I; V, *Eco*RV.

TABLE 2   Staphylococcal plasmids [a]

Type/family/plasmid	Determinant(s) [b]	Size (kb)
Small		
pT181	*tetA*(K)	4.4
pC221	*cat*	4.6
pS194	*str*	4.5
pC194	*cat*	2.9
pSK89	*smr*	2.4
pSK108	*smr*	2.4
pUB110	*aadD, ble*	4.5
pSN2	—	1.3
pSK3	—	1.3
pE194	*ermC*	3.7
pSK639	*dfrA*	8.0
pSK697	*dfrA, smr*	11.0
pSK818	*dfrA, tetA*(K)	13.0
Multiresistance		
β-lactamase family		
pI524 (α)	*arsBC, blaZ, cadA, merAB*	31.8
pII147 (β)	*arsBC, blaZ, cadA, cadB, merAB*	32.6
pI258 (γ)	*arsBC, blaZ, cadA, ermB, merAB*	28.2
pSK23 (α/β)	*aacA–aphD, cadA, merAB, qacB*	38.0
pSK57 (α/γ)	*blaZ, cadA, merAB, qacA*	28.8
pSK1 family		
pSK1	*aacA–aphD, dfrA, qacA*	28.4
pSK4	*aacA–aphD, blaZ, dfrA, qacA*	35.1
pSK18	*qacA*	18.9
Unclassified		
pIP630	*vat, vga, vgb*	22.7
pUL5050	*msrA, blaZ, tet*	31.5
Conjugative		
pSK41 family		
pCRG1600	*aacA–aphD, aadD, blaZ, smr*	52.9
pGO1	*aacA–aphD, aadD, dfrA, smr*	52.0
pGO400	*mupA*	34.0
pJE1	*aacA–aphD, aadD, dfrA, smr*	50.0
pSK41	*aacA–aphD, aadD, smr*	47.8
pUW3626	*aacA–aphD, aadD, blaZ, smr*	54.4
Unclassified		
pIP1156	*vatB, dfrA, blaZ, linA*	60.0
pJ3358	*tetA*(K), *mupA*	34.2

[a]For original references, see Paulsen et al (1996).
[b]Genetic nomenclature as per Table 1.

TABLE 3 Staphylococcal transposons[a]

Element (related)	Size (kb)	Determinant(s)[b]	Associated IS[c]
Tn551	5.3	ermB	NA
Tn552 (Tn4002, Tn4201)	6.1	blaZ	NA
Tn554	6.7	ermA, spc	NA
Tn3854	4.5	?	?
Tn4001 (Tn4031)	4.7	aacA–aphD	IS256
Tn4003	4.7	dfrA	IS257
Tn4291	7.5	mecA	IS257
Tn5404	16	aphA-3, aadE	NA[c]
Tn5405[d]	12	aphA-3, aadE	IS1182[e]

[a]For original references, see Paulsen et al (1996).
[b]Genetic nomenclature as per Table 1.
[c]NA, not associated with any IS element; ?, unknown.
[d]Tn5405 is located entirely within Tn5404.
[e]One copy of IS1182 in Tn5405 contains a copy of IS1181.

integrate formation. Our sequence analyses have now confirmed that, in addition to the pUB110-derived *aadD* portion, at least two other IS257 delimited regions of pSK41 correspond to small plasmid co-integrates (Fig. 2A), including the segment encoding the antiseptic and disinfectant resistance determinant, *smr* (formerly (*qacC/D*) (N. Firth, S. Apisiridej, A. Hettiaratchi, C. D. Scaramuzzi & R. A. Skurray, unpublished data).

Similarly, we have characterized two plasmids, pSK697 and pSK818, that are closely related to the Tp[r] plasmid, pSK639 (Fig. 1), but also contain a co-integrated copy of a second small plasmid and additional flanking copy of IS257 (Leelaporn et al 1996). pSK697 contains a molecule closely related to the CNS *smr*-bearing plasmid, pSK108, whereas pSK818 is co-integrate with a pT181-like *tetA* (K) plasmid; in both cases 8 bp repeats juxtapose the flanking IS257 copies.

The apparent incidence of such IS257-flanked small co-integrated plasmids within other replicons suggests that co-integrate formation represents an important aspect of the activities associated with this element. Indeed, the prevalence of directly repeated copies of IS257 is consistent with the sequential acquisition of resistance determinants via co-integration of target molecules mediated by pre-existing IS257 elements on the capturing replicon. Assembly of multiresistance gene clusters represents an obvious by-product of such behaviour.

Replicon fusions involving IS257 are thought to result from either homologous recombination between a pre-existing element on each of the participating replicons (possibly following replicative transposition of one element from one replicon to the other)(Matthews et al 1990, Thomas & Archer 1989) or co-integration as a direct outcome of IS257 transposition (replicative transposition without resolution) (Byrne

A

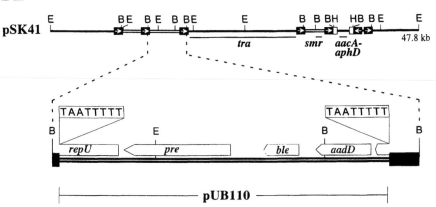

B

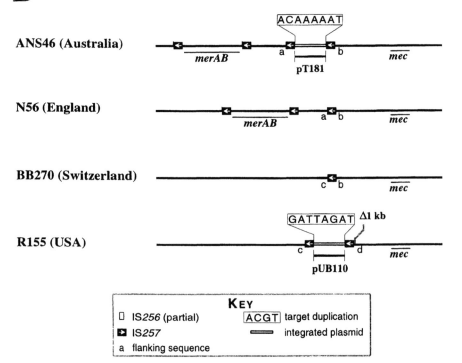

TABLE 4 Antimicrobial resistance determinants associated with IS*257*

Determinant[a]	Location(s)	Reference
aacA–aphD	pSK41 family conjugative plasmids	Byrne et al 1990a
aadD	pSK41 family conjugative plasmids	Byrne et al 1991
	Chromosome	Dubin et al 1991
dfrA	pSK1 family multiresistance plasmids	Rouch et al 1989
	pSK41 family conjugative plasmids	Leelaporn et al 1994
	pSK639 small family plasmids	Leelaporn et al 1994
mecA	Chromosome	Stewart et al 1994
merA, merB	β-lactamase family multiresistance plasmids	Gillespie et al 1987
	Chromosome	Stewart et al 1994
mupA	pSK41 family conjugative plasmids	Morton et al 1995
	Unclassified conjugative plasmid (pJ3358)	Needham et al 1994
smr	pSK41 family conjugative plasmids	Littlejohn et al 1991
	pSK639 small family plasmid (pSK697)	Leelaporn et al 1996
tetA (K)	pSK639 small family plasmid (pSK818)	Leelaporn et al 1996
	Unclassified conjugative plasmid (pJ3358)	Needham et al 1994
	Chromosome	Stewart et al 1994
vgb	Unclassified multiresistance plasmid (pIP630)	El Solh et al 1990

[a]Genetic nomenclature as per Table 1.

et al 1991, Stewart et al 1994). However, the generation of replicon-inactivating insertions (Table 5) would seem more likely to occur in a single co-integration step rather than via transposition followed by homologous recombination, since both of these low-frequency events would have to occur before the replication-defective target plasmid was lost. Furthermore, the fact that 'simple' replicative transposition (i.e. with resolution) of IS*257* has yet to be demonstrated, and the apparent scarcity of individual elements flanked by potential target duplications, suggests that co-integration, or more correctly, replicative transposition without resolution, may represent the typical

FIG. 2. (*opposite*) IS*257*-associated determinants in the conjugative plasmid pSK41 (A), and the chromosomal *mec* region of various methicillin-resistant *S. aureus* (MRSA) isolates (B). In A, an expanded physical and genetic map of the co-integrated copy of pUB110 is shown below the map of pSK41. In B, the country of isolation for each MRSA strain is shown. Target duplications for pSK41 are taken from Byrne et al (1991), whereas the target duplication and flanking sequences for the MRSA chromosomes are taken from Stewart et al (1994). Symbols, abbreviations and layout are as per Fig. 1.

TABLE 5   Small co-integrated plasmids[a]

Determinant	Location(s)	Prototype plasmid	Comments
aadD	pSK41	pUB110	rep insertion
aadD	Chromosome	pUB110	Altered aad regulation
dfrA	pSK1	pSK639 (CNS)	rep deletion
dfrA	pJE1	pSK639 (CNS)	rep deletion
smr	pSK41	pSK89	Deletion of nick site
smr	pSK697 (CNS)	pSK108 (CNS)	Intact
tetA(K)	pJ3358	pT181	Altered rep regulation
tetA (K)	Chromosome	pT181	Altered tet regulation
tetA(K)	pSK818 (CNS)	pT181	rep insertion

[a]Genetic nomenclature as per Table 1 or text. For references, see Table 4.

outcome of IS257 transposition, as has been suggested for the related element IS15 (Trieu-Cuot & Courvalin 1985). Indeed, IS257-mediated co-integration has recently been demonstrated in the laboratory, confirming the transpositional proficiency of the element (Needham et al 1995), although the results obtained do not discriminate between the two potential co-integration modalities. It should be stressed however, that even if IS257 transposition normally occurs without resolution, this does not preclude the possibility that rearrangements can result from homologous recombination between IS257 elements.

IS257 as a portable promoter

The composite transposon-like structure, Tn4003, confers high-level trimethoprim resistance via the dfrA gene which encodes the Tp^r S1 dihydrofolate reductase (DHFR) (Rouch et al 1989). On the S. aureus pSK1 family plasmids, such as pSK4 (Fig. 1), Tn4003 is flanked by a single copy of IS257 at one end (IS257L) and two copies at the other (IS257R1 and IS257R2). In Tn4003, the −35 sequence of the promoter responsible for transcription of dfrA is encoded within the terminal inverted repeat of IS257L, and is teamed with a −10 sequence encoded within the central region (Fig. 3) (Leelaporn et al 1994). Deletions adjacent to the IS257 copy upstream of dfrA that remove the −10 sequence lower the transcriptional activity of the region dramatically and result in a commensurate reduction in the level of trimethoprim resistance expressed, demonstrating the requirement of this promoter for the high-level resistance phenotype (Leelaporn et al 1994).

The recognition of a sequence with the potential to act as an outwardly facing −35 sequence at each end of IS257 has led us to investigate the possibility that IS257-

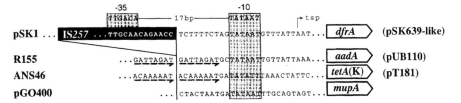

FIG. 3. IS257-derived hybrid promoters. Sequences shown are from the plasmids pSK1 (Rouch et al 1989) and pGO400 (Morton et al 1995), and the chromosomes of the MRSA strains, R155 and ANS46 (Stewart et al 1994). Sequences corresponding to the −35 and −10 consensus sequences are indicated, as is the transcriptional start point (tsp) mapped for Tn4003 on pSK1 (Leelaporn et al 1994). The determinants transcribed from the respective hybrid promoters are shown on the right along with the probable co-integrated plasmids that encode them (if known). The solid box represents the relevant IS257 copy from Tn4003 with the terminal sequence, containing the −35 motif, indicated. The positions of IS257 in the sequences of R155, ANS46 and pGO400 are indicated by the black vertical line. Target duplications are indicated by dashed arrows.

derived hybrid promoters might direct transcription of other genes in a fashion analogous to *dfrA* on Tn4003. Sequence analysis has revealed three candidates where the previously identified IS257-encoded −35 sequence is situated with an appropriately located −10-like sequence, upstream of an antibiotic resistance gene (Fig. 3); viz., the co-integrated pUB110-derived *aadD* in the chromosome of *S. aureus* strain R155 (Fig. 2B; Table 5)(Stewart et al 1994), the co-integrated pT181-derived *tetA*(K) in the chromosome of *S. aureus* strain ANS46 (Fig. 2B; Table 5)(Stewart et al 1994), and *mupA* in the conjugative plasmid, pGO400 (Fig. 1) (Morton et al 1995). In these three cases the resistance determinant is the first gene following the potential promoter, each of which possesses optimal spacing (17 bp) between −35 and −10 boxes. Furthermore, the putative promoters upstream of *aadD* and *mupA* contain a perfect match to the −10 consensus whereas that of *tetA*(K) possesses only a single mismatch (Fig. 3). It is therefore tempting to speculate that these as yet experimentally untested IS257 hybrid promoters may influence the expression of the respective downstream antibiotic resistance genes.

Since target duplications are evident at the termini of the co-integrated copies of pUB110 and pT181 being discussed here (Figs 2 and 3), it would appear that the putative promoters have been formed upon transpositional insertion of IS257 rather than via an IS257-associated adjacent deletion (but see below) akin to those described previously in some pSK639 family plasmids (Leelaporn et al 1994). This observation raises the possibility that such fortuitously located insertions may be selected as a consequential response to facilitate higher levels of resistance. In this regard it is worth considering that in the cases where we can extrapolate the sequence of the target progenitor (the co-integrated copies of pUB110 and pT181), the −10 boxes

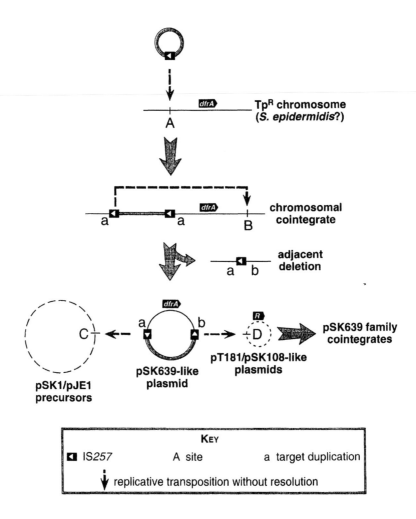

FIG. 4.   Model for the evolution of staphylococcal trimethoprim resistance plasmids. The
details of the model are described in the text. Continuous thin and thick lines denote
chromosomal and plasmid DNA, respectively, whereas thin dashed lines represent target
plasmid DNA. IS257 copies are shown as solid boxes containing arrowheads which indicate
the orientation of the element. Arrowed lines denote replicative transposition without
resolution of the relevant IS257 element into the indicated target site (uppercase); the resulting
target duplications are shown in lowercase. The positions and orientations of resistance genes are
indicated by solid arrowed boxes; *dfrA* encoding S1 DHFR; R, *tetA* (K) in the case of pT181 and
smr in pSK108.

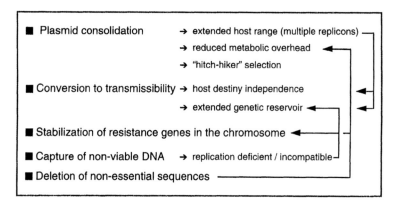

FIG. 5. Outcomes of co-integration. The points are discussed in the text.

identified here were probably not associated with an appropriately positioned − 35-like sequence prior to IS257 insertion.

Role of IS257 in the acquisition and dissemination of trimethoprim resistance

The chromosomal gene encoding the Tp^s (trimethoprim susceptible) DHFR of a coagulase-negative organism, *S. epidermidis* strain ATCC 14990, has recently been sequenced and found to share extensive similarity to *dfrA* in both sequence and flanking genetic organization, implicating this or a closely related species as the origin of the Tp^r variant encoded by Tn4003 and related elements (Dale et al 1995). Tp^r plasmids from CNS may therefore represent the vectors responsible for dissemination of Tp^r among staphylococci (Leelaporn et al 1994). Consistent with this notion, analyses of pSK639 family plasmids isolated from CNS suggest that the Tn4003-like structures identified in *S. aureus* may represent remnants of co-integrated pSK639-like plasmids that have suffered IS257-mediated adjacent deletions. The exclusive association between *dfrA* and copies of IS257 observed to date argues for the involvement of this element in the capture of a chromosomal gene encoding a Tp^r DHFR.

We have devised a model for the evolution of *dfrA*-containing structures in *S. aureus* amended from that proposed by Rouch et al (1989) to incorporate recent findings (Fig. 4). Importantly, this model can accommodate all such structures so far characterized in staphylococci via a single recombinogenic mechanism, viz., replicative transposition of IS257 without resolution. The model also illustrates how the various properties of IS257 contribute to the development of antimicrobial resistance. As illustrated in Fig. 4, only two events are required to liberate the Tp^r determinant from the chromosome. Firstly, IS257 transposition from a 'donor' plasmid into the chromosome adjacent to *dfrA* (site A, Fig. 4); it is conceivable that this insertion resulted in the generation of the

IS257 hybrid promoter upstream of *dfrA* as described above, possibly contributing to increased levels of trimethoprim resistance. A second transposition event, of the more distal resulting element into an opposing site (site B, Fig. 4), would result in two discrete products (Fig. 4). This second event is equivalent in nature to the first, differing only in that the same molecule is both donor and target, and results in two products. One product is a circular molecule (pSK639-like plasmid; Fig. 4), consisting of the intervening segment between the donor element and its target site, which in this case represents a hybrid of the original plasmid and a formerly chromosomal DNA segment containing *dfrA*, separated by directly repeated copies of IS257. This product is structurally analogous to pSK639, which, it should be remembered is mobilizable, a property that may have contributed greatly to the dissemination of high-level Tp^r after liberation of *dfrA* from the chromosome. The other product corresponds to a chromosomal deletion of the intervening segment with an IS257 element at the junction of the deletion endpoints. This product serves to demonstrate how replicative transposition without resolution into the same molecule in direct orientation can account for the adjacent deletions commonly associated with IS257 (Leelaporn et al 1994). Subsequent transposition events by the IS257 elements of such a pSK639-like plasmid into pSK108 and pT181 would result in the co-integrate CNS plasmids pSK697 and pSK818, respectively. Similarly, a co-integration event followed by an adjacent deletion, both mediated by the IS257 elements present on the pSK639-like plasmid, are all that are required to accommodate the Tn4003-like structures present on pSK1 family multiresistance plasmids and the conjugative plasmid pJE1 (Fig. 1).

Conclusions

As a recombinogenic mechanism in the context of antimicrobial resistance, replicative transposition without resolution carries a number of significant ramifications. A summary of several, which also illustrates their inter-relationships, is presented in point form in Fig. 5. The most obvious of these is the assembly of gene clusters, as manifest by the sequential capture of small plasmids as described above. The consolidation of resistance determinants on a single plasmid is expected to contribute to the maintenance of non-selected genes under the imposition of a selection for only one of the resistance determinants encoded by that plasmid ('hitch-hiker' selection); incorporation of determinants in the host chromosome would likewise afford enhanced segregational stability. Similarly, the accretion of antimicrobial resistance genes on conjugative or mobilizable plasmids facilitates the co-transfer on non-selected determinants. This tendency toward transmissibility also avails a plasmid some independence from the destiny of its immediate host and opens the door to the capture (collection?) of additional activities as it moves through different populations; these potentialities are further enhanced by the acquisition of multiple replicons thereby providing an extended host range. Co-integration also provides a means of acquiring determinants present on non-replicative DNA that might be introduced into a cell via any of the gene transfer mechanisms acting in staphylococci.

The net result of these eventualities, which are by no means restricted to IS257-associated co-integrative events, is a greater likelihood of acquisition, maintenance and dissemination of resistance determinants from an extended gene pool. The presence of identical determinants and plasmids in *S. aureus* and CNS testifies to genetic exchange between these groups, and suggests the latter, which includes normally commensal species, may act as a reservoir of resistance genes for the former (Lyon & Skurray 1987). Furthermore, the presence of, for example, Tn*4001*-like gentamicin resistance transposons in enterococci (Hodel-Christian & Murray 1991) and streptococci (de Cespèdes et al 1994), highlight intergeneric transfer mechanisms at work.

Acknowledgements

Work in the laboratory of R.A.S. on staphylococcal resistance is supported by grants from the National Health and Medical Research Council (Australia).

References

Byrne ME, Gillespie MT, Skurray RA 1990a Molecular analysis of a gentamicin resistance transposon-like element on plasmids isolated from North American *Staphylococcus aureus* strains. Antimicrob Agents Chemother 34:2106–2113

Byrne ME, Littlejohn TG, Skurray RA 1990b Transposons and insertion sequences in the evolution of multiresistant *Staphylococcus aureus*. In: Novick RP (ed) Molecular biology of the staphylococci. VCH, New York, p 165–174

Byrne ME, Gillespie MT, Skurray RA 1991 4′,4″ adenyltransferase activity on conjugative plasmids isolated from *Staphylococcus aureus* is encoded on an integrated copy of pUB110. Plasmid 25:70–75

Dale GE, Broger C, Hartman PG et al 1995 Characterization of the gene for the chromosomal dihydrofolate reductase (DHFR) of *Staphylococcus epidermidis* ATCC 14990: the origin of the trimethoprim-resistant S1 DHFR from *Staphylococcus aureus*? J Bacteriol 177:2965–2970

de Cespèdes G, Derbise A, Trieu-Cuot P, Horaud T 1994 Mobile chromosomal elements (Tn*3706* and Tn*3707*) in *Streptococcus agalactiae* B128 resistant to gentamicin and tetracyclines. In: Totolian A (ed) Pathogenic streptococci: present and future. Lancer, St Petersburg, p 272–273

Dubin DT, Matthews PR, Chikramane SG, Stewart PR 1991 Physical mapping of the *mec* region of an American methicillin-resistant *Staphylococcus aureus* strain. Antimicrob Agents Chemother 35:1661–1665

El Solh N, Allignet J, Loncle V, Mazodier P 1990 Nucleotide sequence of a staphylococcal plasmid gene *vgb* encoding a hydrolase that inactivates the B components of virginiamycin-like antibiotics. In: Novick RP (ed) Molecular biology of the staphylococci. VCH, New York, p 617–622

Evans J, Dyke KG 1988 Characterization of the conjugation system associated with the *Staphylococcus aureus* plasmid pJE1. J Gen Microbiol 134:1–8

Firth N, Ridgway KP, Byrne ME et al 1993 Analysis of a transfer region from the staphylococcal conjugative plasmid pSK41. Gene 136:13–25

Gillespie MT, May JW, Skurray RA 1986 Detection of an integrated tetracycline resistance plasmid in the chromosome of methicillin-resistant *Staphylococcus aureus*. J Gen Microbiol 132:1723–1728

Gillespie MT, Lyon BR, Loo LSL, Matthews PR, Stewart PR, Skurray RA 1987 Homologous direct repeat sequences associated with mercury, methicillin, tetracycline and trimethoprim resistance determinants in *Staphylococcus aureus*. FEMS Microbiol Lett 43:165–171

Hodel-Christian SL, Murray BE 1991 Characterization of the gentamicin resistance transposon Tn*5281* from *Enterococcus faecalis* and comparison to staphylococcal transposons Tn*4001* and Tn*4031*. Antimicrob Agents Chemother 35:1147–1152

Leelaporn A, Firth N, Byrne ME, Roper E, Skurray RA 1994 Possible role of insertion sequence IS*257* in dissemination and expression of high-level and low-level trimethoprim resistance in staphylococci. Antimicrob Agents Chemother 38:2238–2244

Leelaporn A, Firth N, Paulsen IT, Skurray RA 1996 IS*257*-mediated cointegration in the evolution of a family of staphylococcal trimethoprim resistance plasmids. J Bacteriol 178:6070–6073

Littlejohn TG, DiBernardino D, Messerotti LJ, Spiers SJ, Skurray RA 1991 Structure and evolution of a family of genes encoding antiseptic and disinfectant resistance in *Staphylococcus aureus*. Gene 101:59–66

Lyon BR, Skurray R 1987 Antimicrobial resistance of *Staphylococcus aureus*: genetic basis. Microbiol Rev 51:88–134

Matthews PR, Inglis B, Stewart PR 1990 Clustering of resistance genes in the *mec* region of the chromosome of *Staphylococcus aureus*. In: Novick RP (ed) Molecular biology of the staphylococci. VCH, New York, p 69–83

Morton TM, Eaton DM, Johnston JL, Archer GL 1993 DNA sequence and units of transcription of the conjugative transfer gene complex (*trs*) of *Staphylococcus aureus* plasmid pGO1. J Bacteriol 175:4436–4447

Morton TM, Johnston JL, Patterson J, Archer GL 1995 Characterization of a conjugative staphylococcal mupirocin resistance plasmid. Antimicrob Agents Chemother 39:1272–1280

Murphy E 1988 Transposable elements in *Staphylococcus*. In: Kingsman AJ, Chater KF, Kingsman SM (eds) Transposition. Cambridge University Press, Cambridge, p59–89

Needham C, Rahman M, Dyke KGH, Noble WC 1994 An investigation of plasmids from *Staphylococcus aureus* that mediate resistance to muriprocin and tetracycline. Microbiol 140:2577–2583

Needham C, Noble WC, Dyke KGH 1995 The staphylococcal insertion sequence IS*257* is active. Plasmid 34:198–205

Novick RP 1989 Staphylococcal plasmids and their replication. Ann Rev Microbiol 43:537–565

Paulsen IT, Firth N, Skurray RA 1996 Resistance to antimicrobial agents other than β-lactams. In: Archer GL, Crossley K (eds) The staphylococci in human disease. Churchill Livingstone, New York, p 175–212

Rouch DA, Skurray RA 1989 IS*257* from *Staphylococcus aureus*: member of an insertion sequence superfamily prevalent among gram-positive and gram-negative bacteria. Gene 76:195–205

Rouch DA, Messerotti LJ, Loo LS, Jackson CA, Skurray RA 1989 Trimethoprim resistance transposon Tn*4003* from *Staphylococcus aureus* encodes genes for a dihydrofolate reductase and thymidylate synthetase flanked by three copies of IS*257*. Mol Microbiol 3:161–175

Shalita Z, Murphy E, Novick RP 1980 Penicillinase plasmids of *Staphylococcus aureus*: structural and evolutionary relationships. Plasmid 3:291–311

Stewart PR, Dubin DT, Chikramane SG, Inglis B, Matthews PR, Poston SM 1994 IS*257* and small plasmid insertions in the *mec* region of the chromosome of *Staphylococcus aureus*. Plasmid 31:12–20

Thomas WD Jr, Archer GL 1989 Mobility of gentamicin resistance genes from staphylococci isolated in the United States: identification of Tn*4031*, a gentamicin resistance transposon from *Staphylococcus epidermidis*. Antimicrob Agents Chemother 33:1335–1341

Trieu-Cuot P, Courvalin P 1985 Transposition behaviour of IS*15* and its progenitor IS*15*-delta: are cointegrates exclusive end products? Plasmid 14:80–89

DISCUSSION

Summers: I noticed especially the multiple IS*257* insertion elements, because they are all potential sites for recombination that could lead to the elimination of resistance determinants. I wonder if you have had a chance to study this?

Skurray: We have yet to do the laboratory experiment where a plasmid-carrying strain is grown and the various progeny are analysed for potential deletions. However, the outcome of such can be seen in the clinical situation; among a series of patient isolates, one can detect a range of deleted plasmids carrying variations of the original plasmid that have presumably arisen through homologous recombination between IS*257* sequences that flank the segment that is deleted. What also remains to be shown is the exact mechanism(s) by which co-integrates between plasmids form. As I described, there are two models of co-integration; one is by replicative transposition without resolution, the other by homologous recombination between two pre-existing insertion sequences, such as IS*257*. We have designed experiments to attempt to distinguish between these two models and to formally demonstrate IS*257* transposition. Dr Keith Dyke at Oxford has carried out an experiment showing IS*257* is active but this was with a recombination-proficient host (Needham et al 1995).

Summers: One wonders how many different possibilities there are. It is conceivable that with a substrate like this you might get some interesting varieties that will tell you something about the mechanisms that might be involved in the field.

Noble: The experiment Ron mentioned arose from observations we made where, from three patients in a ward at the same time, we recovered three different mupirocin resistance plasmids (Needham et al 1994). The simplest had one mupirocin gene flanked by IS*257*, the next had two mupirocin genes, each flanked with IS*257*s and the third one had a complete pT181 integrated, again flanked. There was some evidence that a duplication of the IS*257* was occurring *in situ* and the integration was into that site. The eight base pair repeats at the ends of the IS*257* sequences were identical, which would not happen if an exogenous IS*257* was coming in. This appeared, therefore, to be plasmid evolution in the ward.

Levy: Is this event unique to *S. aureus* because people have looked for it in *S. aureus*, or is it unique to *S. aureus* because this is what the organism likes to do? Are there limited numbers of plasmids that can be maintained in *S. aureus*?

Skurray: No. *S. aureus* is able to accept a wide range of plasmids. Indeed, 15 different incompatibility groups of staphylococcal plasmids have been identified, implying an equivalent number of different replicons. Also, when we talk of clinically significant staphylococci we must not ignore the coagulase-negative staphylococci (CNS); anyone who has looked at the plasmid profiles of CNS strains will know that a single strain may have up to 10 different plasmid types co-existing in the one cell. In some of the latter, different genes giving similar resistance phenotypes may occur together in one cell but be located on different plasmid types; we have seen this with the *qac* genes for antiseptic and disinfectant resistance in a number of CNS strains from Australian hospitals (Leelaporn et al 1994).

Davies: Going beyond that, since *Staphylococcus* spp. are human commensals, you might expect to find global dissemination of similar types of staphylococcal plasmids. Is this seen?

Skurray: Yes. We see similar plasmids in strains from widely separated locations; for example, the pSK41-type conjugative plasmids have been detected in isolates from the USA and from Europe. However, there is also dissemination of similar or identical strains; for example, the so-called 'Australian' MRSA strains have been detected in England.

Levy: How much of the resistance is clonal and how much is it plasmid spread? We've been led to believe that MRSA is relatively clonal.

Skurray: Yes, there does appear to be a high degree of clonality among many MRSA strains. However, even these related MRSA have been separated into at least six different allied groups depending on hybridization patterns with methicillin-resistant *mec* region DNA, and some of these sub-groups could be further divided on the basis of patterns with the chromosomal transposon Tn*554* as probe, suggesting there may have been various polymorphic rearrangements in the MRSA chromosome subsequent to the acquisition of the *mec* gene (Kreiswirth et al 1993).

Hall: In terms of subdivisions of *mec*-containing strains, do people still argue that originally there was one *mec* acquisition event and that these subdivisions are subsequent events?

Skurray: Yes. This was the argument made by Kreiswirth et al (1993).

Hall: What is your opinion?

Skurray: As you know, it is very difficult to make absolute statements about the temporal acquisition and spread of resistance genes such as *mec*, which first emerged in *S. aureus* some 35 years ago; we can only make best guesses based on the strains we have available in our retrospective collections. However, given this, it does seem that although many MRSA strains are clonal, the *mec* region has been acquired on more than one occasion and that this was to *S. aureus* strains of different backgrounds or lineages (Musser & Kapur 1992). This has also been argued by Dr Keiichi Hiramatsu from Tokyo on the basis of ribotyping and analysis of the genetic organization of the *mec* regions of epidemic strains he collected from around the world (Hiramatsu 1995). Also, it has been suggested that one of the routes of transfer of the *mec* region to *S. aureus* has been via a CNS species, such as *S. haemolyticus* (Archer et al 1994).

Witte: There is some evidence that the *mec* gene jumped to quite different groups of strains. Dr Hiramatsu has sequenced the 40 kb *mec*-associated DNA which is always associated with the *mec* gene. He has found three or four different sequence groups. I recall the multilocus enzyme work performed by Dr Musser showing that five different clonal groups of MRSA exist. We have analysed other chromosomal polymorphisms by microrestriction profiling and have seen the *mec* gene in one strain of the clonal group which is able to produce toxic shock syndrome toxin and in another clonal group which is also spread outside hospitals and sensitive to methicillin.

We do not know on which mechanisms the staphylococcal carrier stage is based. But these multiply resistant staphylococcal hospital strains are not disseminated by nasal carriers in the community. With carriers of MRSA who have left the hospital, we have not seen it spread in their families.

Levy: Could the corollary then be that the evolution of these strains has occurred in the hospital? You did mention the use of topical antibiotics.

Skurray: Yes. There is no doubt in my mind that the extensive use of topical antibiotics represents a significant selective force in the hospital environment leading to the emergence and maintenance of resistance. Also antibiotics in the hospital environment may actually promote the transfer of resistance among bacteria by conjugation or other means.

Levin: We have done jointly theoretical and experimental studies of the evolution of multiple resistance plasmids. In an article by Rick Condit and myself (Condit & Levin 1990), we demonstrate that if complementary resistance genes are borne on separate, incompatible plasmids and both antibiotics are used, single plasmids carrying both resistance genes (or alternative stable situations, such as the movement of one resistance gene onto the chromosome) will evolve at a rapid rate due to selection against segregants that lose one or other resistance gene. Currently, Peter Sykora and I are working on the situation where the complementary resistance genes are borne on pairs of compatible plasmids, variants of R100 (Cm) and Sa (Km). When we allow for the transfer of these plasmids to a plasmid-free recipient and select for transconjugants with both the Cm and Km markers, a major fraction of these two marker transconjugants are co-integrates for the Sa and R100 plasmids.

Hall: Both of those plasmids have an integron. Consequently they both possess an integrase and you would expect integrase-mediated co-integration. R100 also has transposons and ISs, and these can also cause co-integrate formation. It is actually quite easy to map them and show where the recombination events occurred—then you know for sure.

Levin: Right on Ruth. It looks like a Tn*21* is associated with that co-integration process with an integrase mechanism very much like you describe. These *in vitro* evolution studies make me wonder how many naturally occurring R plasmids have been formed by analogous co-integration mechanisms and thus how many naturally occurring multiple resistance (and other) plasmids are chimeras derived from two or more plasmids.

Hall: Like staphylococci, many Enterobacteriaceae have multiple plasmids but people haven't examined this in much detail, so there is only old literature. There are also cases where what is clearly a single plasmid has two integrons. One simple mechanism for achieving this is exactly as you have described, by the formation of a co-integrate.

Levin: The R100–1-Sa co-integrate plasmid that evolved in Peter Sykora's and my experimental evolution studies appears to be stable. Neither segregants nor single marker resistance plasmids were observed among the 200 or so colonies we tested after maintaining these bacteria in antibiotic-free culture for more than 50 generations.

Summers: We looked at a bunch of human strains collected from the Boston area in the early 1980s. We concentrated on a subset of about 59 mercury-resistant ones and 22 mercury-sensitive ones. Roughly 90% of the mercury-resistant ones had an integron (unpublished results).

Levy: How common are the integrates? We reported a co-integrate plasmid from a clinical *E. coli* strain isolated in Indonesia (Bradley et al 1986). The clinical isolate had a single plasmid with co-integrated plasmids from two incompatibility groups.

Hall: Many plasmids are made up of several discrete components. If you take R100, which is probably the most-studied large multidrug resistance plasmid out of the original Watanabe collection, the bits that have been identified as being transposons constitute quite a lot of it. This is also true for the mercury resistance plasmid pVS1. Of about 30 kb, most is accounted for by Tn*501* and the integron In*0*. Only a few kb are left, and the replication and stability regions take up at least 1 kb. You see transposons and then more transposons inside the transposons. That the transposons actually tend to pile up inside one another is probably because the bits of the original plasmid in between them are required for other functions, such as replication, stability and transfer.

Levy: What is the basis of the integration of plasmid pT181?

Skurray: As I commented previously, it is most likely based on co-integrative transposition or what might be more accurately described as non-resolved transposition. A single copy of IS*257* present on one replicon, say the chromosome, would have transposed to pT181 by replicative transposition, forming a co-integrate molecule between the plasmid and the chromosome which is not resolved.

Levy: To summarize then, there are many interesting ways in which plasmids can be built up and strains can become more resistant. These mechanisms are probably not present just for resistance, but they're being elicited for that purpose. In the staphylococci, especially, there is an obvious model of building up resistance. How large can the multiple resistance become and why don't these plasmids start losing the resistance genes? They seem to be remarkably stable. For instance, the staphylococci do not appear to be losing their antiseptic resistance despite decreased use of antiseptics.

Skurray: That's a lovely example to comment on. Firstly, the antiseptic resistance *qac* and *smr* genes also give resistance to a wide range of disinfectant compounds which are still in common use, namely quaternary ammonium compounds, dyes and biguanidines; the *qac*/*smr* genes encode multidrug resistance export or efflux proteins which reduce the intracellular levels of the compound (Paulsen et al 1996). Secondly, although the level of resistance that these genes give is insufficient for a cell carrying them to withstand high concentrations of directly applied antiseptics and disinfectants, such cells may well be able to survive the residual levels of these toxic compounds that remain in a hospital environment. Thirdly, since the *qac/smr* genes are frequently carried on multiresistance plasmids, such as the pSK1 family or the pSK41 family of conjugative plasmids that I described, these residual levels of antiseptics/disinfectants would provide a selective pressure not only for the maintenance of the *qac/smr* genes but also for the many other determinants carried on these plasmids (see Fig. 1). This would be a very nice case of 'hitch-hiker' selection.

Noble: There are two recent examples, one from Australia (Udo et al 1994) and one from America (Morton et al 1995), where a pre-existing plasmid carrying genes for resistance to penicillin in one case and gentamicin in the other had those genes replaced by a mupirocin resistance determinant, but the rest of the plasmid stayed intact. This reminded me of the 'plasmid addiction' which we mentioned earlier, where a strain gets fixed with its tetracycline resistance plasmid and can't manage without.

Roberts: Haemophilus influenzae started out with a large R plasmid carrying Amp^r. During the 1970s other antibiotic resistance genes were added and some were removed. The antibiotic resistance genes had been rearranged and most of the rest of the plasmid had been left intact. No one has looked since the 1970s, but in the 7–10 years after the introduction of antibiotic resistance in 1973, one plasmid type was rearranged with new antibiotic resistance genes.

Levin: In at least the short term, associated linkage selection will play an important role in the maintenance of resistance to antibiotics no longer in use. This is probably the reason for the high frequency of resistance to streptomycin Bassam Tomeh observed in his studies of antibiotic resistance among the faecal flora of children in a day-care centre. Next to ampicillin resistance, and I expect resistance to other β-lactam antibiotics as well, streptomycin resistance was the most frequent resistant marker we observed among the bacteria obtained from the faecal flora of these infants. As I understand it, streptomycin is rarely used clinically.

Cohen: But it is used in the environment, for example, as a spray on fruit trees.

Hall: The streptomycin resistance determinant in the resistant *Erwinias* from Californian fruit trees is also found in human isolates.

Levy: But there has to be a reason why it has remained. We can still ask, why do bacteria have plasmids? The plasmids were there before antibiotics became extensively used. When we talk about stability of resistances, we are really looking at ancient vehicles, plasmids that have been around for a long time. Ron Skurray, you have sequenced entire staphylococcal plasmids. Are there any genes on some of the larger plasmids that might be beneficial to the host apart from resistance determinants?

Skurray: We have not detected any genes on these large staphylococcal plasmids that might be of benefit to the host other than the resistance determinants, but there are a number of open reading frames for which we have no function at present. However, I don't think we should focus too much on the question of why plasmids exist. Rather, the more important questions concern why so many resistance genes are captured and maintained so successfully in the staphylococci: i.e. what are the most important selective pressures? Also, where have these genes been acquired from? That is, what are the origins of resistance genes and how extensive is the staphylococcal gene pool?

Roberts: The 2.6 cryptic *Neisseria gonorrhoeae* plasmid has been found in over 90% of all isolates. It has been completely sequenced. There are four open reading frames, nobody has a clue why it's there, and there's really no difference between those strains that do and don't have the plasmid.

Lenski: One explanation is that conjugative plasmids don't need to provide a benefit to the host cell if they make their living as a sort of a weak parasite, one that imposes very little burden on its host and has enough horizontal transmission to maintain itself in the system (Levin & Lenski 1983). As an alternative hypothesis, Ron Skurray emphasized the building up of more and more complex plasmids: clearly that happens, but the maintenance of a non-conjugative plasmid might occur by the decay of a plasmid to the point that it does no harm to its host. Paul Turner (1995) has done experiments in which non-conjugative plasmids evolved from a conjugative plasmid. The non-conjugative plasmids may have a long half-life in the population because they're causing no harm to the bacteria, even though they are not actually beneficial. So, under conditions where there's a lot of opportunity for plasmid transfer, the plasmid may make a living by moving at a sufficiently high rate to offset any harm done to its host, while under other conditions a non-conjugative plasmid may sit around for a very long time simply because it's doing so little harm that it will take a long time to disappear from the population.

Levin: Most *E. coli* we isolated from natural populations carried one, and usually more than one plasmid of unknown function — so-called cryptic plasmids (see e.g. Caugant et al 1981). The composition and structure of these accessory elements may well be the most variable element of the *E. coli* genome. One of my former students, Lin Lin Fu, surveyed this cryptic plasmid variation among strains of *E. coli* isolated from urinary tract infections studied by Catharina Svanorg and her colleagues. All of these strains were obtained over a two year period from school girls in Gothenberg, Sweden. Nevertheless, among strains with identical 20 enzyme ETs and the same specific O:K:H ET strains from different sources, Lin Lin was able to find restriction fragment variation in these plasmids.

Hall: I can't see any reason why not.

Davies: I thought these origin of replication regions were all different.

Levin: If co-integration is a common mechanism, we are going to find multiple origin of replication regions in the same plasmid.

Summers: Co-integration doesn't happen at the origin of replication, anyway.

Levin: But you are forming a double plasmid.

Skurray: In many cases the co-integration event has led to a deletion or an insertion in one of the replicons, thereby inactivating that replicon. In other cases, co-integration may well lead to an enhanced expression of resistance; the latter likely occurs with IS257 which carries the −35 sequence of a promoter within it's terminal inverted repeat (see Fig. 3).

Summers: We're looking at 'hot house' cases here because most of us are talking about what happens with strains that have been isolated from patients in the context of multiple resistance. We know far too little about larger populations and what is going on with these plasmids in bacteria generally when they just come out of the normal flora of non-hospitalized persons.

Baquero: Are there any historical isolates of *S. aureus* we could look at to see whether these sequences were present in isolates before antibiotics were used? The machinery *S. aureus* has used to become multiply resistant was probably already present to enable adaptation to the changing environments in different animals. The process has probably only been accelerated by the use of antibiotics.

Levy: In evolution, you can go from point A to point B, but when you get to point B other things happen that mean that you can't go back to point A. Some would say it is selection on the outside that is keeping it the way it is. On the other hand, if we could get rid of that selection, will the bacterium go back to a susceptible state? It is interesting that those studies haven't been done, because this will determine how we deal with MRSA. If staphylococcus is a new creature with multidrug resistance, how will we deal with it if it gains vancomycin resistance?

Lenski: I want to give some sense on how long it would take to lose something that has a cost, but a very small cost. Imagine a population size in the order of 10^9 bacteria. Then introduce a single mutant that gets rid of some unnecessary function that imposes a 10% cost. It will take more than 250 generations for that single mutant to become the majority type in the population. If there is only a 1% cost, it's going to take more than 2500 generations. If it has only a 0.1% cost, you're going to have to run the experiment for more than 25 000 generations to see the mutant that has lost the useless function become the predominant type.

Levy: That's an example of how a plasmid-bearing strain may lose the plasmid. If you introduce into that environment some other organism, it may well take over.

Davies: Richard, do you know of other cases of regressive evolution where a gene acquired by a bacterial strain has been lost?

Lenski: When we did the experiment on coadaptation of *E. coli* and pACYC184 (Bouma & Lenski 1988), we tried first to do it in a chemostat without any antibiotic selection. But the plasmid was quickly lost because it reduced the fitness of the bacteria so much that spontaneous plasmid-free segregants eliminated the plasmid-bearing cells (Lenski & Bouma 1987).

We have done another relevant experiment that doesn't involve antibiotic resistance. We used a single strain of *E. coli* to start 12 replicate lines that we propagated in a minimal glucose medium for several years. The bacteria went through 10 000 generations (Lenski & Travisano 1994). We're just now starting to ask how much the bacteria have eliminated unused metabolic functions. For instance, can they still metabolize lactose, which they haven't used for 10 000 generations? My first impression is that there has been very little regressive evolution over that period. One of the reasons may be that many of these genes are regulated, so there's only the marginal cost of carrying that little extra bit of

DNA, which is probably very cheap if the bacteria is not actually transcribing the message or producing the protein. That leads to a question concerning MRSA: are the antibiotic resistance genes regulated?

Davies: Aminoglycoside resistance is constitutively expressed in all bacterial strains tested to date.

Baquero: It's possible to accelerate the loss of a trait that only has a slight cost if you put these strains in competition with others.

Cohen: It might be interesting to compare nosocomial and community-acquired staphylococci. Over the last couple of years I've seen several instances in which penicillin-susceptible staphylococci have caused community-acquired infections. I'm curious as to whether or not there may be different trends in nosocomial and community-acquired staphylococci.

Gaynes: I do not think so. I haven't seen a penicillin-susceptible *S. aureus* from a community-acquired infection in 15 years.

Lerner: I encountered penicillin-susceptible *S. aureus* in an intravenous drug user with endocarditis. It was weird to treat *S. aureus* endocarditis with penicillin G, but I believed the susceptibility test results and indeed the patient was cured.

Noble: I have looked at 800 *S. aureus* from the community sent in by GPs to the lab. 96% produced penicillinase; the other resistances were really quite low: 11% were resistant to tetracycline, 6% resistant to erythromycin, 3% resistant to fusidic acid and only one strain of the 800 was resistant to anything else.

References

Archer GL, Niemayer DM, Thanassi JA, Pucci MJ 1994 Dissemination among staphylococci of DNA sequences associated with methicillin resistance. Antimicrob Agents Chemother 38:447–454

Bouma JE, Lenski RE 1988 Evolution of a bacteria/plasmid association. Nature 335:351–352

Bradley DE, Taylor DE, Levy SB, Cohen DR, Brose EC, Whelan J 1986 pIN32: a co-integrate plasmid with IncHI2 and IncFII components. J Gen Microbiol 132:1339–1346

Caugant DA, Levin BR, Selander RK 1981 Genetic diversity and temporal variation in the *Escherichia coli* population of a human host. Genetics 98:467–490

Hiramatsu K 1995 Molecular evolution of MRSA. Microb Immunol 39:531–543

Kreiswirth B, Kornblum J, Arbeit RD et al 1993 Evidence for a clonal origin of methicillin resistance in *Staphylococcus aureus*. Science 259:227–230

Leelaporn A, Paulsen IT, Tennent JM, Littlejohn TG, Skurray RA 1994 Multidrug resistance to antiseptics and disinfectants in coagulase-negative staphylococci. J Med Microbiol 40:214–220

Lenski RE, Bouma JE 1987 Effects of segregation and selection on instability of pACYC184 in *Escherichia coli* B. J Bacteriol 169:5314–5316

Lenski RE, Travisano M 1994 Dynamics of adaptation and diversification: a 10 000 generation experiment with bacterial populations. Proc Natl Acad Sci USA 91:6808–6814

Levin BR, Lenski RE 1983 Coevolution in bacteria and their viruses and plasmids. In: Futuyama DJ, Slatkin M (eds) Coevolution. Sinauer Associates, Sunderland, MA, p 99–127

Morton TM, Johnston JL, Patterson J, Archer GL 1995 Characterization of a conjugative staphylococcal mupirocin resistance plasmid. Antimicrob Agents Chemother 39:1272–1280

Musser JM, Kapur V 1992 Clonal analysis of methicillin-resistant *Staphylococcus aureus* from intercontinental sources: association of the *mec* gene with divergent phylogenetic lineages implies dissemination by horizontal transfer and recombination. J Clin Microbiol 30:2058–2063

Needham C, Rahman M, Dyke KGH, Noble WC 1994 An investigation of plasmids from *Staphylococcus aureus* that mediate resistance to mupirocin and tetracycline. Microbiology 140:2577–2583

Needham C, Noble WC, Dyke KGH 1995 The staphylococcal insertion sequence IS*257* is active. Plasmid 34:198–205

Paulsen IT, Firth N, Skurray RA 1996 Resistance to antimicrobial agents other than β-lactams. In: Archer GL, Crossley K (eds) The staphylococci in human disease. Churchill Livingstone, New York, p 175–212

Turner PE 1995 Associations between bacteria and conjugative plasmids: model systems for testing evolutionary theory. PhD thesis, Michigan State University, East Lansing, MI, USA

Udo EE, Pearman JW, Grubb EB 1994 Emergence of high level mupirocin resistant *Staphylococcus aureus* in Western Australia. J Hosp Infect 26:157–165

Mobile gene cassettes and integrons: moving antibiotic resistance genes in Gram-negative bacteria

Ruth M. Hall

CSIRO, Division of Biomolecular Engineering, Sydney Laboratory, PO Box 184, North Ryde, NSW 2113, Australia

Abstract. In Gram-negative pathogens, multiple antibiotic resistance is common and many of the known resistance genes are contained in mobile gene cassettes. Cassettes can be integrated into or deleted from their receptor elements, the integrons, or infrequently may be integrated at other locations via site-specific recombination catalysed by an integron-encoded recombinase. As a consequence, arrays of several different antibiotic resistance genes can be created. Over 40 gene cassettes and three distinct classes of integrons have been identified to date. Cassette-associated genes conferring resistance to β-lactams, aminoglycosides, trimethoprim, chloramphenicol, streptothricin and quaternary ammonium compounds used as antiseptics and disinfectants have been found. In addition, most members of the commonest family of integrons (class 1) include a sulfonamide resistance determinant in the backbone structure. Integrons are themselves translocatable, though most are defective transposon derivatives. Integron movement allows transfer of the cassette-associated resistance genes from one replicon to another or into another active transposon which facilitates spread of integrons that are transposition defective. Horizontal transfer of the resistance genes can be achieved when an integron containing one or more such genes is incorporated into a broad-host-range plasmid. Likewise, single cassettes integrated at secondary sites in a broad-host-range plasmid can also move across species boundaries.

1997 Antibiotic resistance: origins, evolution, selection and spread. Wiley, Chichester (Ciba Foundation Symposium 207) p 192–205

Resistance to antibiotics leading to failure of antibiotic therapy for bacterial pathogens was first encountered shortly after the introduction of antibiotics. Since then resistance to antibiotics has inevitably emerged in response to the introduction of new or modified antibiotics, though the time taken has varied. Because resistance to many antibiotics does not arise by mutation of the bacterial chromosome, but rather by the acquisition of new genes whose products effect resistance by a variety of mechanisms, the study of antibiotic resistance (particularly in Gram-negative bacteria) has led to a number of discoveries that have had substantial impact on our understanding of bacterial genomes and how they evolve (Davies 1995). The first of these was the discovery in the early 1960s of the 'resistance transfer factors' (RTFs), which are examples of the small extra-chromosomal genomes now commonly known as plasmids. Furthermore, many plasmids, including the RTFs, can be transferred from one cell to another and in some cases across species boundaries (horizontal gene transfer). A second important concept is that of transposition, i.e. movement of discrete genetic units (insertion sequences and transposons) from one location to another, and particularly from one genome to another. The discovery of these translocatable elements revealed that genomes are far more plastic than was previously thought, and provided an explanation for how plasmids could capture new genes.

The ability of Gram-negative bacteria to acquire antibiotic resistance genes and subsequently to spread them to many bacterial species was largely but not completely explained by plasmids and transposons. Resistance genes present in transposons could move onto various plasmids, and once present on a plasmid which was transfer-proficient could spread from one bacterium to another. If the plasmid also had the ability to be transferred to and maintained in more than one bacterial species, horizontal transfer to new species could also occur. However, the way in which transposons acquire resistance genes was not fully understood. A resurgence of interest in bacterial antibiotic resistance over the last decade has led to the somewhat belated sequencing of many antibiotic resistance genes and, as a consequence, the discovery of a novel system for the movement of antibiotic resistance genes. This system is comprised of an already large family of discrete mobile genetic units called gene cassettes that each contain only one (antibiotic resistance) gene, and a family of receptor elements — integrons — that provide both the site into which gene cassettes are integrated and the enzyme responsible for gene movement. Movement of gene cassettes, i.e. their integration into and excision from integrons, is effected by site-specific recombination. Recent reviews (Hall & Collis 1995, Recchia & Hall 1995a) include more detail and more extensive referencing. However, integrons are also translocatable and this feature is clearly important in the movement of resistance genes across species boundaries as it permits integrons and the resistance genes they carry to become associated with a variety of broad-host-range plasmids. This aspect of the dissemination of resistance genes found in mobile gene cassettes is also addressed.

Mobile cassettes containing antibiotic resistance genes

Many of the antibiotic resistance genes found in Gram-negative bacterial pathogens are part of discrete genetic units known as gene cassettes (see Hall et al 1991, Recchia & Hall 1995a for compilations). The genes confer resistance to many different antibiotics, aminoglycosides, trimethoprim, chloramphenicol, penicillins and cephalosporins, and for each of these antibiotic families several distinct resistance genes have been found in gene cassettes (Table 1). Single examples of genes conferring resistance to quaternary ammonium compounds used as antiseptics and to the antibiotic streptothricin, which

TABLE 1 Gene cassettes encoding antibiotic resistance genes

Gene cassette and gene[a]	Protein[b]	Activity	Class of family[c]
Resistance to β-lactams			
blaP1	CARB-2 (PSE-1)	β-lactamase	A
	CARB-3, PSE-4		
blaP2	—	β-lactamase	A
blaP3	CARB-4	β-lactamase	A
bla$_{IMP}$	IMP-1	β-lactamase	B
oxa1	OXA-1, OXA-8, OXA-4	β-lactamase	D
oxa2	OXA-2	β-lactamase	D
oxa3	OXA-3	β-lactamase	D
oxa5	OXA-5	β-lactamase	D
oxa7	OXA-7	β-lactamase	D
oxa9	OXA-9	β-lactamase	D
oxa10	OXA-10 (PSE-2),	β-lactamase	D
	OXA-11, OXA-14		
Resistance to aminoglycosides			
aadA1a	AAD(3″)	Aminoglycoside (3″) adenylyltransferase	1
aadA1b	AAD(3″)	Aminoglycoside (3″) adenylyltransferase	2
aadA2	AAD(3″)	Aminoglycoside (3″) adenylyltransferase	3
aadB	AAD(2″)	Aminoglycoside (2″) adenylyltransferase	
aacA1	AAC(6′)-Ia	Aminoglycoside (6′) acetyltransferase	1
aacA4	AAC96′)-Ib, AAC(6′)-IIc	Aminoglycoside (6′) acetyltransferase	2
aacA (orfB)	AAC(6′)-Id	Aminoglycoside (6′) acetyltransferase	3
aacA7	AAC(6′)-II	Aminoglycoside (6′) acetyltransferase	3
aacA	AAC(6′)-IIa	Aminoglycoside (6′) acetyltransferase	2

Gene	Protein	Description	Family
aacA	AAC(6')-IIb	Aminoglycoside (6') acetyltransferase	2
aacC1	AAC(3)-Ia	Aminoglycoside (3) acetyltransferase	
aacC	AAC(3)-Ib	Aminoglycoside (3) acetyltransferase	

Resistance to chloramphenicol

Gene	Protein	Description	Family
catB2	CATB2	Chloramphenicol acetyltransferase	B
catB3	CATB2	Chloramphenicol acetyltransferase	B
catB5	CATB5	Chloramphenicol acetyltransferase	B
cmlA	CmlA	Chloramphenicol exporter	

Resistance to trimethoprim

Gene	Protein	Description	Family
dfrA1	DHFRIa	Dihydrofolate reductase	A
dfrA5	DHFRV	Dihydrofolate reductase	A
dfrA7	DHFRVII	Dihydrofolate reductase	A
dfrA12	DHFRXII	Dihydrofolate reductase	A
dfrA13	DHFRXIII	Dihydrofolate reductase	A
dfrA14	DHFRIb	Dihydrofolate reductase	A
dfrB1	DHFRIIa	Dihydrofolate reductase	B
dfrB2	DHFRIIb	Dihydrofolate reductase	B
dfrB3	DHFRIIc	Dihydrofolate reductase	B

Resistance to streptothricin

Gene	Protein	Description
sat	SAT-2	Streptothricin acetyltransferase

Resistance to antiseptics and disinfectants

Gene	Protein	Description
qacE	QacE	Quaternary ammonium compounded exporter

[a] Sources of cassette sequences and locations of cassettes and genes are found in Recchia and Hall (1995b). Cassettes are named after the gene they encode. However, in many cases the genes have not previously been assigned names and in some cases, the gene nomenclature used here differs from that found in the original publications. As an agreed numbering system for the *aacA* and *aacC* genes is not currently available, several of these genes are not numbered.

[b] Where more than one protein name is listed the nucleotide sequences are identical (brackets) or differ at fewer than 5 positions. Variations in *oxa10* and *aacA4* cause changes in the resistance spectrum.

[c] Protein families include enzymes that are significantly related (> 20–25% identity). The *dfrA* and *dfrB* genes encode dihydrofolate reductase proteins belonging to two distinct families. For the aminoglycoside resistance determinants, products of the *aadA* and *aacC* genes listed are related, and families are indicated only for the *aacA* genes which determine acetyltransferases from three distinct families.

is not used in human therapy, have also been identified. To date over 40 cassettes have been identified by sequencing (Table 1, compiled in Recchia & Hall 1995a) and many more are likely to be found in the future. All but five of the known cassettes contain resistance genes.

Gene cassettes form a family of mobile elements that are quite distinct from transposons. Each cassette includes only a single gene and a recombination site (59 base element) that is located downstream of the gene and confers mobility (Fig. 1A). Cassettes differ from transposons in that they are not bounded by inverted repeats and do not encode the enzyme responsible for their movement.

Cassette movement

Cassette movement is catalysed by a site-specific recombinase, IntI, that is encoded by an integron (Fig. 1B; see below). The recombinase belongs to the integrase family exemplified by λ integrase (Ouellette & Roy 1987) and recognises specific sites, the 59 base element in a cassette and the *attI* site in an integron. A single conservative site-specific recombination event results in the integration of a circular gene cassette into an integron (Collis et al 1993) and the reverse reaction leads to excision of the cassette in a circular form (Collis & Hall 1992a,b). The uptake of one cassette does not preclude the uptake of further cassettes and, as a consequence, arrays of several cassettes each containing a different resistance gene can be created (Fig. 1C).

Integrons: the receptors for gene cassettes

Integrons contain a recombination site, designated *attI*, that acts as the receptor site for the gene cassettes and also encode the catalytic machinery, namely the IntI integrase. A further function supplied by the integrons is a promoter that is required for expression of the genes in the integrated cassettes (Fig. 1C). The need for this common promoter arises from the fact that the vast majority of cassettes do not include a promoter, and when more than one integrated cassette is present in an integron the cassette genes are co-transcribed (Collis & Hall 1995).

Three distinct classes of element that include all three of the features (integrase gene, receptor site and promoter) that define integrons have so far been found (see Hall et al 1991, Recchia & Hall 1995a); these are described in more detail below. Class 1 includes the majority of the integrons found in clinical isolates to date, and only members of this class were originally named integrons (Stokes & Hall 1989). Class 1 integrons have been most extensively studied and have been used in all of the experimental studies of cassette movement published to date.

Members of each integron class have identical or nearly identical integrases, but quite distinct integrases (40–60% amino acid identity) are encoded by each of the three classes (Hall & Vockler 1987, Arakawa et al 1995). Somewhat surprisingly, despite the differences in the sequences of the integrases and the *attI* sites, the same gene cassettes appear to be able to be taken up by all three integron classes, as

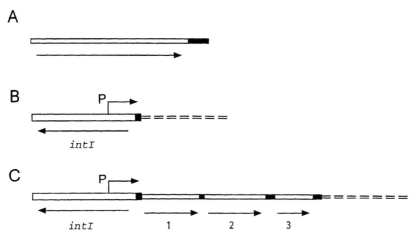

FIG. 1.   Structure of gene cassettes and integrons. A representative gene cassette (A), an integron (B), and an integron containing three integrated cassettes (C) are shown. For the gene cassettes, the filled area shows the extent of the 59 base element recombination site and the arrow indicates the extent of the gene, assuming that the first in-frame initiation codon is used. A similar configuration of *intI* gene and *attI* site (filled box) and promoter (P) for expression of genes in integrated cassettes is found in integrons belonging to classes 1, 2 and 3. However, known class 2 integrons (Tn7 and relatives) contain a mutation in the *intI* gene that creates an in-frame stop codon (see Hall & Vockler 1987, Recchia & Hall 1995a).

identical cassettes have been found in class 1 and class 2 integrons (Hall et al 1991, Sundström & Sköld 1990) or in class 1 and class 3 integrons (Arakawa et al 1995).

Other integrase-mediated reactions

Potentially the most important further reaction catalysed by the IntI1 integrase is recombination between one specific site and a secondary site. Though secondary sites are recognized only very inefficiently, this type of reaction has been observed experimentally (Francia et al 1993, Recchia et al 1994). Such events can potentially lead to the integration of cassettes at many positions outside integrons and one case in which the *aadB* gene cassette has been precisely incorporated into a plasmid closely related to the broad-host-range IncQ plasmid RSF1010 has been documented (Recchia & Hall 1995b). Though in this case the cassette-associated recombination site is inactivated by the integration event (Recchia & Hall 1995b), further studies have revealed that in some cases an active recombination site is regenerated (G. D. Recchia & R. M. Hall, unpublished data). When this occurs the site can presumably act as a target for further cassette integration events and cassette arrays could then be created at such locations.

Recombination events between two IntI-specific recombination sites, that are equivalent to those that lead to integration and excision of circular cassettes into and from integrons, and events involving one specific and one secondary site equivalent to those described above, can also lead to rearrangements of the genomes of plasmids that contain integrons (see Hall & Collis 1995, Recchia & Hall 1995b for detailed descriptions). In this case, the first reaction leads to formation of a co-integrate; subsequent excision events can, if they involve a different pair of sites, give rise to rearrangements or reassortment of the features present in two different plasmids contained in the same cell.

Integron mobility

Integrons of class 1 are mobile, but have diverse structures that are described below. Class 2 includes the transposon Tn7 and a number of close relatives (see Hall et al 1991, Recchia & Hall 1995a). Tn7 includes three integrated cassettes adjacent to a defective integrase gene located at the left end. Only a single example of class 3 has been found so far (Arakawa et al 1995) and at this stage it is not known if class 3 integrons are also translocatable.

Although class 1 integrons are found in many different locations on plasmids, within transposons such as Tn21 and in bacterial chromosomes, only one member of this class is known to be an active transposon. A recent report of the complete sequence of Tn402 (Rådström et al 1994) revealed that this transposon is a class 1 integron. In addition to the integrase module and three integrated cassettes, Tn402 includes a set of four putative transposition genes (Fig. 2) that are presumed to be required for transposition, by analogy with the closely related genes in Tn5053 which have been studied experimentally (Kholodii et al 1995).

However, the vast majority of class 1 integrons that have been examined to date appear to be highly rearranged transposition-defective derivatives of a Tn402-like ancestor. These integrons generally contain the *sul1* gene, conferring resistance to sulphonamides, that is found in a conserved DNA segment (3'-conserved segment) located downstream of the integrated cassettes. This region is present only in class 1 integrons but is not present in Tn402, implying that it was acquired prior to the spread of the *sul1*-containing class 1 integrons. Three integrons of this type have now been completely sequenced, and the sequences of substantial regions of three further examples have also been determined (Hall et al 1994, Brown et al 1996, H. J. Brown, G. D. Recchia, H. W. Stokes & R. M. Hall, unpublished observations). Two groups of *sul1*-containing integrons with distinctive structures were found (Fig. 2). Members of the first group retain part of the Tn402 transposition gene (*tni*) module, but include the insertion sequence IS1326. IS1326 appears to have caused deletions that extend for different distances into the 3'-conserved segment and *tni* module (Brown et al 1996). Members of the second group retain only 154 bases from the outer end of the *tni* module and contain the insertion sequence IS6100. In both groups the loss of transposition genes has created defective transposon derivatives. However, because the outer ends of the original transposon, including the terminal 25 bp inverted repeats, are retained (Rådström et al 1994, Hall et al 1994), these derivatives should

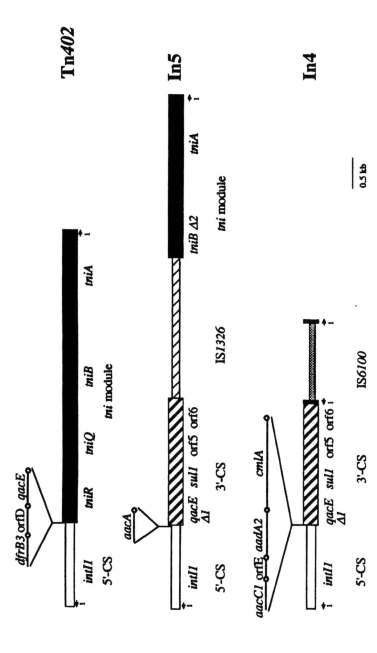

FIG. 2. Structures of class 1 integrons. Representatives of the three types of backbone structure found amongst class 1 integrons are shown. The 5'-CS (*intI* module) is an open box and the integrated cassettes are shown above. The 3'-CS is represented by a diagonally hatched box, and transposition (*tni* genes) module by a filled box. Insertion sequences present in In5 and In4 are hatched and stippled, respectively.

be able to move if transposition proteins are supplied *in trans* by a related transposon in the same cell.

Class 1 integrons located within transposons

Class 1 integrons that are themselves defective transposons are sometimes found within other active transposons, the best known example being Tn*21* which contains the integron In2. The insertion of a class 1 integron into a transposon that is a member of the Tn*21* subgroup of the Tn*3* transposon family has occurred on at least three independent occasions to give rise to Tn*21*, Tn*1696* and Tn*1403*. Each of these transposons has a different backbone structure and contains an intergron located at a different position (Hall et al 1994, G. D. Recchia, H. J. Brown, H. W. Stokes and R. M. Hall, unpublished observations). Tn*21* and its closest relatives are derived, by various insertion and deletion events, from a common ancestor that had acquired an integron (Brown et al 1996). The movement of an integron that has lost its own transposition functions into another active transposon has clear advantages for the spread of that integron. This is evidenced by the fact that Tn*21* and other transposons of this family were first found in the multidrug-resistant *Shigella* strains isolated in Japan in the 1950s, and related transposons continue to be prevalent in multidrug-resistant bacteria to the present day.

Host range and horizontal gene transfer

The antibiotic resistance genes contained in mobile gene cassettes have been found in many bacterial species including *Escherichia, Shigella, Salmonella, Morganella, Klebsiella, Enterobacter, Acinetobacter* and *Pseudomonas,* indicating that inter-species transfer of integrons and gene-cassettes has been a common occurrence. In order for horizontal transfer of an antibiotic resistance gene to occur, the gene must first be taken up by the new host and then stably maintained. The simplest way in which this can be achieved is if the gene first becomes associated with a broad-host-range plasmid that carries conjugation functions or is mobilizable. The fact that integrons are themselves translocatable elements is clearly important in this regard, as it permits them to move into such plasmids. Indeed, class 1 integrons have been found in several broad-host-range plasmids such as R46 (IncN), R388 and pSa (IncW) and R751 (IncP1). However, horizontal transfer of single genes can also be achieved by the direct integration of a mobile gene cassette at a secondary site in a broad-host-range plasmid; this is the case for the *aadB* cassette in found in an RSF1010 derivative (IncQ). Finally, it is possible that gene cassettes in their free circular form could be sufficiently stable to survive cell lysis and be taken up by a new host by transformation. If this host contains an integron and hence an IntI integrase, it would be possible for the cassette to become integrated either within the integron or elsewhere.

Conclusions

The many different resistance genes found in gene cassettes are very efficiently packaged as mobile genetic units that can be readily acquired by integrons and also integrated at other sites. Gene cassettes represent a new class of mobile elements that move by site-specific recombination. Integrons and gene cassettes are found in many Gram-negative bacterial species, belonging to the Enterobacteriaceae family and *Pseudomonas* genus and this wide distribution has presumably been achieved by transposition of integrons to broad-host-range plasmids. A few integrons are transposons but most of the integrons found in clinical isolates are defective remnants of transposons that have intact outer ends and so can move only when transposition functions are supplied *in trans*. In some cases, integrons that are themselves defective transposons have enhanced their mobility by moving into other active transposons. Overall, the picture that has emerged is one of patchwork genomes; integrons (transposons) that carry one or several gene cassettes, composite transposons that carry one or more further transposons (including integrons) within them and plasmids that carry one or more transposons each containing one or more antibiotic resistance genes. The ability of integrons to take up more than one cassette encoding an antibiotic resistance determinant, the association of integrons with larger transposons that may carry further antibiotic resistance genes and the association of multiple transposons with the same plasmid, together explain the common occurrence of bacterial strains that are simultaneously resistant to many different antibiotics. The existence of these plasmids argues for caution before widely using antibiotics — even those not used in human therapy — in animal husbandry, aquaculture and horticulture.

References

Arakawa Y, Murakami M, Suzuki K et al 1995 A novel integron-like element carrying the metallo β-lactamase gene bla_{IMP}. Antimicrob Agents Chemother 39:1612–1615

Brown HJ, Stokes HW, Hall RM 1996 The integrons In0, In2 and In5 are defective transposon derivatives. J Bacteriol 178:4429–4437

Collis CM, Hall RM 1992a Site-specific deletion and rearrangement of intergron insert genes catalysed by the integron DNA integrase. J Bacteriol 174:1574–1585

Collis CM, Hall RM 1992b Gene cassettes from the insert region of integrons are excised as covalently closed circles. Mol Microbiol 6:2875–2885

Collis CM, Hall RM 1995 Expression of antibiotic resistance genes in the integrated cassettes of integrons. Antimicrob Agents Chemother 39:155–162

Collis CM, Grammaticopoulos G, Briton J, Stokes HW, Hall RM 1993 Site-specific insertion of gene cassettes into integrons. Mol Microbiol 9:41–52

Davies J 1995 Vicious circles: looking back on resistance plasmids. Genetics 139:1465–1468

Francia MV, de la Cruz F, García Lobo M 1993 Secondary sites for integration mediated by the Tn21 integrase. Mol Microbiol 10:823–828

Hall RM, Collis CM 1995 Mobile gene cassettes and integrons: capture and spread of genes by site-specific recombination. Mol Microbiol 15:593–600

Hall RM, Vockler C 1987 The region of the IncN plasmid R46 coding for resistance to β-lactam antibiotics, streptomycin/spectinomycin and sulphonamides is closely related to antibiotic resistance segments found in IncW plasmids and in Tn21-like transposons. Nucleic Acids Res 15:7491–7501

Hall RM, Brookes DE, Stokes HW 1991 Site-specific insertion of genes into integrons: role of the 59-base element and determination of the recombination cross-over point. Mol Microbiol 5:1941–1959

Hall RM, Brown HJ, Brookes DE, Stokes HW 1994 Integrons found in different locations have identical 5′ ends but variable 3′ ends. J Bacteriol 176:6286–6294

Kholodii GY, Mindlin SZ, Bass IA, Yurieva OV, Minakhina OVSV, Nikiforov VG 1995 Four genes, two ends, and a res region are involved in transposition of Tn5053: a paradigm for a novel family of transposons carrying either a mer operon or an integron. Mol Microbiol 17:1189–1200

Ouellette M, Roy PH 1987 Homology of ORFs from Tn2603 and from R46 to site-specific recombinases. Nucleic Acids Res 15:55

Rådström P, Sköld O, Swedberg G, Flensburg J, Roy PH, Sundström L 1994 Transposon Tn5090 of plasmid R751, which carries an integron, is related to Tn7, Mu, and the retroelements. J Bacteriol 176:3257–3268

Recchia GD, Hall RM 1995a Mobile gene cassettes: a new class of mobile element. Microbiol 141:3015–3027

Recchia GD, Hall RM 1995b Plasmid evolution by acquisition of mobile gene cassettes: plasmid pIE723 contains the aadB gene cassette precisely inserted at a secondary site in the IncQ plasmid RSF1010. Mol Microbiol 15:179–187

Recchia GD, Stokes HW, Hall RM 1994 Characterisation of specific and secondary recombination sites recognised by the integron DNA integrase. Nucleic Acids Res 22:2071–2078

Stokes HW, Hall RM 1989 A novel family of potentially mobile DNA elements encoding site-specific gene-integration functions: integrons. Mol Microbiol 3:1669–1683

Sundström L, Sköld O 1990 The dhfrI trimethoprim resistance gene of Tn7 can be found at sites in other genetic surroundings. Antimicrob Agents Chemother 34:642–650

DISCUSSION

Baquero: What proportion of cassettes contain only open reading frames without apparent function?

Hall: Of the 43 completely sequenced cassettes, there are five without known function. However, we have only looked in a very specific niche: the known cassettes have all been found in resistant clinical isolates, because people have been cloning resistance genes from these. Therefore the only other ORFs that have been found are those sitting next to the resistance genes. Gene cassettes may be an extremely common phenomenon somewhere else in the bacterial world, and the resistance genes may be a very small subset of the total genes found in cassettes.

Baquero: Would it be possible for you to look for these cassettes in environmental isolates by PCR for 59 base elements, for instance?

Hall: Unfortunately 59 base elements are a poor target for PCR. They conform to a consensus but they conform poorly, so there's really no sequence that one can go after as a PCR primer.

Levy: Why not use the *int*?

Hall: Integrons in environmental isolates could be found this way, but not all of them. The integrase gene, *intI1*, which is associated with the integrons that are most common, is now only one of three known *int* genes whose integrases recognize cassettes, and it may in fact transpire that it's only one of many more *int* genes.

Davies: We have found integrase genes in the Murray collection (Davies 1997, this volume) but they do not appear to be associated with antibiotic resistance. So far, we have identified integrases in two out of about 40 different isolates from the collection.

Summers: Are the strains phenotypically sensitive?

Davies: Yes, but we have only tested for resistance to the more common antibiotics.

Spratt: Are there any open reading frames associated with these *int* genes?

Davies: The work is preliminary; we have not generated enough nucleotide sequence to know whether there are genes associated with the integrases. The two integrase-positive strains are *Shigella* spp. isolates from 1918 and 1942—both well before the introduction of antibiotics.

Hall: I would argue from the highly developed nature of the structure of class 1 integrons found in the clinical isolates we study that they had been around for a long time prior to antibiotic use. Already two different ISs had come in and created havoc, and the two evolutionary lines created had separated only after the *sul1* gene had been incorporated. All of this must have happened before they appeared in clinical isolates. Tn*21* contains an evolved class 1 integron from NR1 (also known as R100), which is one of the Watanabe plasmid isolated in Japan in the 1950s. So, the first time that multiple resistance appeared in *Shigella*, this evolved integron structure was there.

What seems to have happened is that this integron emerged through the eye of the selection needle. Then, because it had the very successful characteristic that it had also found its way onto a transposon, i.e. Tn*21*, and because it came out early, it has now spread round the world. Today, Tn*21*-like transposons are one of the common places you find integrons. So finding evidence for class 1 integrons in the Murray collection is very nice because I would have predicted they were out there and the resistance genes simply hijacked the system.

Bush: It is interesting that there are only three class A β-lactamases that are coded on cassettes but there are seven class Ds. However, the class A enzymes have been causing the epidemics. The majority of the class D enzymes have been found in a single isolate, not as the cause for large outbreaks of β-lactam resistant infections.

Hall: That's possibly less true than it appears. Very few hybridization studies have been done. The *oxa* (class D β-lactamases) genes could be frequently present along with the TEM. No one has really looked carefully. In one published study, *oxa1* is quite common and *oxa2* is rare, but we've only sequenced three complete cassette arrays and *oxa2* has turned up in two of them.

Bush: But it is not causing serious clinical problems.

Hall: That may be the case, but certainly it is known that in some Turkish strains mutations in *oxa10* have turned the OXA-10 β-lactamase into a better β-lactamase.

Bush: In the Turkish experience, there is almost always a single isolate, not a major epidemic.

Hall: It's certainly true that the TEMs and the SHVs dominate at present, but that may simply be due to their success in spreading. Though the other cassette-associated genes can move around too, whether they're there is not so important at present because Tn*3* is so successful. However, cassette-associated β-lactamase genes are also quite common and may cause future epidemics. The cassette-associated imipenem resistance gene may turn out to be such a case.

Levy: Karen Bush's point is that there are other ways of moving things around apart from the integron. Still, the integron has clearly helped explain phenomena. It is of importance for attempts to reverse resistance that these integration events are not easily reversible, if at all.

Cohen: In some ways this is reminiscent of immunoglobulin synthesis in higher animals, where there is this facility for moving components around to change immunoglobulin structure.

Concerning the proximity of the genes to the promoter: what happens if you use different selective pressures in experiments where you get such re-organizations?

Hall: When we were doing that work, we used a dose dependent gene that we knew had the identical sequence in two different integrons, but different cassettes were in front of it. The level of resistance that we were getting from those two integron regions cloned in the same vector was different. We began with the one with the low level of resistance and put it under selective pressure for higher level resistance. What we isolated were integrons where the genes in front had dropped out. We got these at high enough frequencies that one would predict it would happen with the number of bacteria that are around in an infection, i.e. there are likely to be rearranged cassette arrays present that could have a selective advantage.

Cohen: So do you think these events are primary deletions?

Hall: We know they were because we sequenced all the boundaries.

Summers: We've seen the same thing. We see a variety of insert sizes, depending upon which antibiotic you use for selection prior to doing PCR.

Hall: In fact there's a lot of things happening in this system constantly at a very low level, so it's in a sense like mutation creating diversity at low frequencies.

Cohen: Is this another potential method one could use to achieve susceptibility? In other words, by the restriction of antibiotics can you actually encourage deletion of the cassettes?

Hall: There you are asking for cassette deletion events to happen at a high frequency, whereas they are like mutations in that they happen at a very low frequency. When selective pressure is applied these rare products of deletion are managing to dominate, whereas when there's no selective pressure they won't, because the probability of them coming up from the very low frequency to being the dominant structure in the population is vanishingly small. Unfortunately, the selective pressure is in the direction of retaining the resistance gene.

Levy: Ola Sköld told us yesterday that trimethoprim resistance comes in multiple determinants, while there are only two forms of sulfonamide resistance, one of which is the *sul1* gene, which is part of the integron. Why is the sulfonamide resistance gene found in an integron? Is it because of historical use, or does it have some feature that aids formation of the integron?

Sköld: Yes, *sul1* occurs in the Tn*21* integron, and could be an incomplete cassette. It lacks the 59 base pair tail in this context, but it could be an ancient cassette. One line of evidence for this is that in Tn*21* it truncates the *qacE* gene and prevents its expression. But in Tn*402* *sul1* is not present, and then the *qacE* is an untruncated cassette which can move as Ruth has mentioned. *Sul1* is also found on remnants of integrons on small plasmids. It is hard to know whether it was originally part of a cassette that moved around.

Levy: What you are saying, then, is that integron remnants are found in *Haemophilus* and *Mycobacterium*, so they are not just limited to the Enterobacteriaceae.

Levin: There's something missing from this picture: the whole dynamics. You are just seeing the end product.

Hall: It's hard to do anything but watch the end product. We would love to have properly preserved strains from the preantibiotic era, or sulfonamide-resistant strains isolated prior to the introduction of further antibiotics.

Levin: You can study this prospectively, if you know what the selective pressures are. We have done this. When we studied the evolution of multiple resistance plasmids we found only a couple of mechanisms in terms of the genetics and population dynamics. I believe these are awesome elements that could have evolved very rapidly.

Hall: The event(s) that lead to a gene becoming part of a gene cassette are likely to be extraordinarily rare. However, once the cassette is formed and it gets into an integron, the gene can move about much more readily.

Spratt: You said that new cassettes always go in at the promoter-proximal end. Does that mean that if you have a large number of cassettes you can work out actually the chronology of how cassettes went in?

Hall: Yes and no. Cassettes definitely go in experimentally at the front, but then there are a whole lot of other events that can happen, such as co-integration and resolution events that alter the cassette order. So it's hard to know.

Summers: For the most highly conserved part of the 59 base element, you can get 90 hits on it in the current database. Most of them are clearly associated with bona fide antibiotic resistance genes, but it is also possible that the element is moving by itself.

Reference

Davies JE 1997 Origins, acquisition and dissemination of antibiotic resistance determinants. In: Antibiotic resistance: origins, evolution, selection and spread. Wiley, Chichester (Ciba Found Symp 207) p 15–35

Genetic mobility and distribution of tetracycline resistance determinants

Marilyn C. Roberts

Department of Pathobiology, Box 357238, School of Public Health and Community Medicine, University of Washington, Seattle, WA 98195-7238, USA

Abstract. Since 1953, tetracycline-resistant bacteria have been found increasingly in humans, animals, food and the environment. Tetracycline resistance is normally due to the acquisition of new genes and is primarily due to either energy-dependent efflux of tetracycline or protection of the ribosomes from its action. Gram-negative efflux genes are frequently associated with conjugative plasmids, whereas Gram-positive efflux genes are often found on small mobilizable plasmids or in the chromosome. The ribosomal protection genes are generally associated with conjugative transposons which have a preference for the chromosome. Recently, tetracycline resistance genes have been found in the genera *Mycobacterium*, *Nocardia*, *Streptomyces* and *Treponema*. The Tet M determinant codes for a ribosomal protection protein which can be found in Gram-positive, Gram-negative, cell-wall-free, aerobic, anaerobic, pathogenic, opportunistic and normal flora species. This promiscuous nature may be correlated with its location on a conjugative transposon and its ability to cross most biochemical and physical barriers found in bacteria. The Tet B efflux determinant is unlike other efflux gene products because it confers resistance to tetracycline, doxycycline and minocycline and has the widest host range of all Gram-negative efflux determinants. We have hypothesized that mobility and the environment of the bacteria may help influence the ultimate host range of specific *tet* genes. If we are to reverse the trend towards increasingly antibiotic-resistant pathogenic bacteria, we will need to change how antibiotics are used in both human and animal health as well as food production.

1997 Antibiotic resistance: origins, evolution, selection and spread. Wiley, Chichester (Ciba Foundation Symposium 207) p 206–222

Tetracyclines are broad-spectrum antimicrobial agents with activity against a wide range of bacterial and protozoan parasites (Chopra et al 1992, Roberts 1996). They have been used extensively to treat bacterial respiratory, periodontal and urogenital tract diseases, rickettsia and Lyme's disease. Tetracyclines were the first major group of antibiotics to which the term 'broad-spectrum' was ascribed. Because of their spectrum of activity, relative safety and low cost, they have been widely used throughout the world in both human and animal medicine. However, their use has declined as bacterial resistance has become more widespread (Chopra et al 1992, Levy 1992, Roberts 1989a, 1994, 1996).

Tetracyclines gain access into the bacterial cell by passive diffusion and an energy-dependent active transport (Chopra et al 1992). They are actively concentrated by most bacterial cells and act as bacteriostatic agents which inhibit growth rather than kill *in vitro* by reversibly binding to the ribosomes and inhibiting protein synthesis. They bind to the bacterial 30S ribosomal subunit and prevent attachment of aminoacyl-tRNA to the ribosomal receptor site (Chopra et al 1992, Roberts 1996).

In 1953, the first tetracycline-resistant bacteria isolated was *Shigella dysenteriae*, which causes bacterial dysentery (Falkow 1975, Watanabe 1963). The first multi-resistant *Shigella*, isolated in 1955, was resistant to tetracycline, streptomycin and chloramphenicol (Falkow 1975, Watanabe 1963), and represented 0.02% of the isolates tested. By 1960, multi-resistant *Shigella* represented almost 10% of the strains tested in Japan (Falkow 1975, Watanabe 1963). In the 1950s the Japanese demonstrated that the antibiotic-resistant *Shigella* could transfer their resistant phenotypes to susceptible isolates by co-cultivation. This transfer was dependent upon direct contact of the bacteria (Watanabe 1963). We now know that these were the first reports of tetracycline-resistant efflux genes carried on conjugative R-plasmids.

Tetracycline resistance is also common in Gram-positive species. A recent study (Goldstein et al 1994) indicated that approximately 90% of methicillin-resistant *Staphylococcus aureus*, 70% of *Streptococcus agalactiae*, 70% of multi-drug resistant *Enterococcus faecalis* and 60% of multi-drug resistant *Streptococcus pneumoniae* now are tetracycline resistant. The published data suggest that tetracycline resistance has become widespread in both Gram-positive and Gram-negative species.

Mendez et al (1980) first examined the genetic heterogeneity of tetracycline resistance determinants from Enterobacteriaceae and Pseudomonadaceae plasmids using restriction enzyme analysis, DNA–DNA hybridization and expression of resistance to tetracycline and various analogues. DNA–DNA hybridization with the structural genes as probes is now the standard method used to distinguish distinct tetracycline resistance (*tet*) genes (Mendez et al 1980, Roberts 1996). A new gene is identified by its inability to hybridize with any of the known *tet* genes under stringent conditions, which indicates < 80% sequence identity. If this is demonstrated, then a letter designation is given (Mendez et al 1980). The structural gene of any class would be designated as *tetA* (P) for the first gene and *tetB*(P) for the second gene as is found in the class P. However, other than Tet P, all other classes of tetracycline resistance determinants so far described carry a single structural gene (Roberts 1994). Currently, 17 different *tet* genes have been identified. Fifteen of the *tet* genes are known to code for either efflux of tetracycline (*tetA–tetE, tetG, tetH, tetK, tetL, tetA*(P)) or protection of the ribosomes to the action of tetracycline (*tetM–tetO, tetB*(P), *tetQ, tetS*). The *tetI* gene most likely codes for an efflux system (Jones et al 1992a, Roberts 1996), though it has not yet been sequenced. The last gene, *tetX*, codes for an enzyme which inactivates tetracycline (Roberts 1994, 1996). This enzyme is novel because it requires oxygen to function, but is found only in strict anaerobes where oxygen is excluded (Roberts 1994) and thus is unlikely to function in its natural hosts.

My laboratory has been interested in looking at the change in the distribution of *tet* genes over time and investigating their spread into new bacterial species and genera from a variety of different ecosystems. We have looked at whether there is a correlation between host range, mobility of various *tet* genes, and environment of the bacteria. We have proposed that the normal flora found in each ecosystem may act as a significant reservoir for these genes and play a role in their spread into new species (Roberts 1989a). The tetracycline efflux and ribosomal protection genes have counterparts in the antibiotic-producing streptomyces and thus could be ancestrally related to the *otr* genes *otrA* and *otrB* which code for either ribosomal protection or efflux proteins, respectively. The study of the *tet* genes has provided insights into evolution, selection and spread of antibiotic resistance genes through bacterial populations.

Mobility and distribution of *tet* determinants

Gram-negative genera

The majority of the Tet determinants are associated with either conjugative or mobilizable elements (Table 1) which may partially explain their wide distribution among bacterial species (Jones et al 1992b, Mendez et al 1980). The host ranges of Gram-negative plasmids have been studied and a number of incompatibility groups defined (Jones et al 1992b, Mendez et al 1980). The Gram-negative efflux determinants are normally found on transposons inserted into a diverse group of plasmids from a variety of incompatibility groups (Jones et al 1992b, Mendez et al 1980). These plasmids may carry multiple antibiotic resistance genes which confer resistance to a number of different classes of antibiotics (Acar et al 1977, Falkow 1977, Jones et al 1992b, Roberts 1989a). Plasmid host ranges vary from very restrictive, such as the

TABLE 1   Location of Tet determinants

Plasmid	*Chromosome*
Tet A–E	Tet B, Tet E (rare)
Tet G–H	
Tet I	
Tet K–L	Tet K, Tet L (rare)
Tet M (some species)	Tet M
Tet O	Tet O
Tet S	Tet S
Tet P	
Tet Q	Tet Q

Tet M, Tet Q and Tet S determinants can be associated with conjugative transposons, making them mobile even when located in a chromosome.

large conjugative *Haemophilus* R-plasmids (Acar et al 1977, Roberts 1989a,b, Watanabe 1963) which do not readily survive outside their own genus, to plasmids with broad host ranges which allow the plasmid to survive in diverse host backgrounds (Acar et al 1977, Falkow 1975). The number of different *tet* genes found in a particular Gram-negative genus varies from one to six *tet* genes, though any one Gram-negative isolate most commonly carries a single gene type (Roberts 1994, 1996).

Thirteen genera carry a single determinant: *Actinobacillus, Moraxella, Treponema, Yersinia* (which carry *tetB* [efflux]); *Alcaligenes* (*tetE* [efflux]); *Eikenella, Kingella, Neisseria* (*tetM* [ribosomal protection]); *Campylobacter* (*tetO* [ribosomal protection]); and *Capnocytopha, Mitsuokella, Prevotella, Porphyromonas* (*tetQ* [ribosomal protection]) (Roberts 1996). In the genus *Vibrio*, six different *tet* efflux genes have been characterized (*tetA–E* and *tetG*) (Roberts 1994, 1996).

Recently, we have shown that both *Actinobacillus actinomycetemcomitans* (Roe et al 1995) and *A. pleuropneumoniae* (Wasteson et al 1996) can carry the *tetB* gene. All three genera (*Actinobacillus, Haemophilus, Pasteurella*) within the group Pasteurellaceae can carry *tetB* (Table 2). Nevertheless, *Haemophilus* spp. may also carry *tetK* or *tetM*, while *Pasteurella* spp. may carry *tetD, tetH*, or *tetM* (Roberts 1994, 1996). We have found that some isolates of the anaerobic oral species *Treponema denticola* carry *tetB* on their chromosome (Table 2) (Roberts et al 1996). *T. denticola* is thought to be associated with periodontal disease and is in the same general environment as *Haemophilus* spp. and *A. actinomycetemcomitans*. However, *Haemophilus* spp. are killed when grown anaerobically with *T. denticola* in the laboratory (Roberts et al 1996). This is the first strictly anaerobic species shown to carry the *tetB* gene (Table 2). We have sequenced the PCR fragment generated from one *T. denticola* and found 90% identity between it and Tn*10* (Roberts et al 1996). The *tetB* genes were located in the

TABLE 2   Distribution of Tet B in Gram-negative genera

Enterobacteriaceae	*Other species*
Citrobacter	*Aeromonas*
Escherichia	*Actinobacillus*
Enterobacter	*Haemophilus*
Klebsiella	*Moraxella*
Salmonella	*Pasteurella*
Shigella	*Plesiomonas*
Serratia	*Treponema*[a]
Proteus	*Vibrio*
Providencia	
Yersinia	

[a]*T. denticola* is a strict anaerobe.

chromosome and were non-mobile in laboratory experiments. However, *T. denticola* isolates could transfer *ermF* genes to recipient *Enterococcus faecalis*, indicating that *T. denticola* is able to participate in conjugation as a donor. The *ermF* gene is on a conjugate transposon in the chromosome (Roberts et al 1996).

Non-mobile chromosomal *tetB* genes have been found in a few *Haemophilus* spp. and *Moraxella catarrhalis* (Roberts 1989b, 1994, Roberts et al 1991). However, this is the exception (Roberts 1996). *tetB* is unique among the efflux genes because the TetB protein confers resistance to tetracycline, doxycycline and minocycline while the other efflux proteins do not confer resistance to minocycline (Chopra et al 1992, Roberts 1996). The *tetE* gene can be found on the chromosome or on large non-conjugative plasmids (Roberts 1996). Of the Gram-negative efflux genes, *tetB* has the widest host range and is found in 18 different Gram-negative genera (Table 2), while *tetA*, *tetC*, *tetD* and *tetE* are found in 12, 10, 11 and 7 genera, respectively (Table 3) (Roberts 1996). Why the *tetB* gene is more widely distributed is not known. The *tetA*, *tetC* and *tetD* genes are found primarily among the enteric genera. The *tetE* gene tends to be found in genera associated with both fresh and seawater and does not appear to be associated with mobile plasmids, thus it is unclear how it moves. Little has been done to examine the distribution of *tetG*, *tetH* or *tetI* genes (Roberts 1996).

The ribosomal protection genes are generally thought to be of Gram-positive origin but are now often found in a variety of aerobic and anaerobic Gram-negative species

TABLE 3   Distribution of Tet determinants

Determinant	Number of genera
Tet A	12
Tet B	18
Tet C	10
Tet D	11
Tet E	7
Tet K	12
Tet L	10
Tet M	15
Tet O	8
Tet S	2
Tet P	1
Tet Q	11
Otr A	2
Otr B	2
Otr C	1

(Roberts 1996). Their presence in natural Gram-negative isolates indicates that gene exchange between Gram-positive and Gram-negative bacteria is possible and does occur in nature. The ribosomal protection gene, *tetO*, can be found on conjugative plasmids, or in the chromosome where it is not self-mobile (Roberts 1996). The *tetM* and *tetQ* genes are generally associated with conjugative chromosomal elements, which code for their own transfer (Clewell et al 1995, Roberts 1996) (Table 1). These conjugative transposons have been shown to transfer mobilizable plasmids and the Tet Q transposons may transfer unlinked genomic DNA (Clewell et al 1995, Li et al 1995, Roberts 1996). *Bacteroides* Tet Q conjugative transposons can range from 65 to over 150 kb, most elements carry both *tetQ* and *ermF*, which codes for an rRNA methylase, and belong to a family of elements with the prototype being Tc^r Em^r DOT (Li et al 1995, Roberts 1996). Tet M transposons can range from 18 to > 50 kb and also may carry other antibiotic resistance genes (Clewell et al 1995). These Tet M multidrug-resistant elements have not been found outside Gram-positive species; more work needs to be done on this issue.

Gram-negative anaerobic species and some non-enteric Gram-negative species such as *Neisseria, Eikenella* and *Kingella* most commonly or exclusively carry ribosomal protection genes (*tetM, tetO, tetQ*) (Roberts 1996). One exception is the genus *Haemophilus*, where all of the isolates of *H. influenzae* and *H. parainfluenzae* described in the literature have been shown to carry the *tetB* efflux gene (Roberts 1989a). However, no recent studies have been done to see if this is as true in 1996 as it was in the 1970s. We have characterized a few isolates of *Haemophilus aphrophilus* from periodontal patients in the 1990s. These isolates can carry the *tetK* gene (Pang et al 1994), while *H. ducreyi* has been found to carry either *tetB* and/or *tetM* genes (Roberts 1989b). We have also characterized a few isolates of *Veillonella parvula* that carry either *tetL* or *tetQ*, although most of the isolates examined carry *tetM* (author's unpublished observations).

There has been little work done to elucidate why some Gram-negative genera carry only a single *tet* gene, whereas members of other genera can carry a variety of different *tet* genes. The mobility of a particular gene certainly plays some role in gene distribution but to what extent is not clear. The environment of a particular bacteria may also influence which genes it carries, especially if the environment is polluted or exposed to antibiotics (Andersen & Sandaa 1994, Levy 1992). More work needs to be done to provide a better understanding of the factors influencing not only whether the bacteria will carry tetracycline resistance, but which and how many determinants will be found in a particular species or genus. Most of the Gram-negative isolates described by my laboratory and the literature carry only a single *tet* gene at any one time, thus an isolate would only carry *tetA* or *tetB* but not both (Jones et al 1992b, Mendez et al 1980, Roberts 1996). In fact, the only study where Gram-negative species were reported in high number to carry more than a single *tet* gene is the recent study of polluted marine sediments from Norway (Andersen & Sandaa 1994). In that study, 26% of tetracycline-resistant isolates carried both Tet D and Tet E determinants, while other studies have normally found < 10% carrying more then a single Tet determinant. This differs from the Gram-positive species which commonly carry multiple different genes for tetracycline resistance (Roberts 1996).

Gram-positive genera

The *tetK* gene is found in 12 genera including one Gram-negative species, while *tetL* is found in 10 genera including one Gram-negative species (Table 3) (Roberts 1996). This is in spite of the fact that *tetK* and *tetL* are generally found on small transmissible plasmids which on occasion become integrated into the chromosome of staphylococci (Gillespie et 1986), the chromosome of *Bacillus subtilis* (Sakaguchi & Shishido 1988), or on larger staphylococcal plasmids (Needham et al 1994). The large staphylococcal plasmids carrying *tetK* are relatively uncommon and may carry other antibiotic resistance genes (Needham et al 1994). In contrast, the small plasmids carrying the *tetK* are common and represent a family of closely related plasmids ranging from 4.35 to 4.7 kb (Projan & Novick 1988). pT181 is the prototype of the family and has been completely sequenced (Khan & Novick 1983). The pT181 family of plasmids can carry antibiotic resistance genes other than *tetK* (Projan & Novick 1988).

The *tetK* and *tetL* genes can be found together in single isolates of clostridium, staphylococci, streptococci, peptostreptococci, mycobacteria and streptomyces (Pang et al 1994a,b, Roberts 1996) and may be found in the same isolate with *tetM*, *tetO*, *tetP*, *otrA*, *otrB* or *otrC* (Table 4). Recently, the host range of these two efflux genes has been extended to include *Mycobacterium* spp., *Nocardia* spp. and *Streptomyces* spp. isolated from humans (Pang et al 1994a,b, Doran et al 1997) (Table 4). This suggests that gene exchange between these genera and classical bacteria, such as the Gram-positive cocci, does occur in nature. The most logical explanation for the presence of *tetK* and/ or *tetL* in streptomyces is that the flow of genes is both from and to the streptomyces. Some of the *Mycobacteria* spp. and *Nocardia* spp. carried the *otrA* and *otrB* genes. This strongly suggests that there is gene exchange between the antibiotic-producing *Streptomyces* and other bacteria.

Not all the Gram-positive and Gram-negative isolates resistant to tetracyclines carry one of the known *tet* or *otr* genes (Roberts 1996) (Table 4). Whether the *tet* and/or *otr* genes are responsible for the resistance phenotype in *Mycobacterium* spp., *Nocardia* spp. and *Streptomyces* spp. that we have examined in Table 4 has not been proven. However, susceptible isolates did not hybridize with any of the gene probes tested (Table 4). The PCR product from *M. avium* ATCC 35712 had 98% sequence identity over 350 bp with *tetK* sequence from *S. aureus*. The PCR product from *M. fortuitum* showed similar sequence identity to *tetK* (Pang et al 1994a,b). The distribution of the *otr* and *tetP* genes has not been extensively examined and may be wider than indicated by Table 3.

The ribosomal protection genes *tetM*, *tetO*, *tetQ* and *tetS* are all found in Gram-positive species (Roberts 1994, 1996). Except for *tetO*, all the other genes are normally associated with conjugative transposons (Clewell et al 1995, Roberts 1996). *tetO* is mobile when associated with conjugative plasmids. Few experiments have looked at the movement of *tetS*. Tet M and Tet Q conjugative elements are hypothesized to involve a Rec-independent excision event which produces a non-replicative circular intermediate that can insert at a different site within the cell or transfer to a new host by a conjugative plasmid-like process (Clewell et al 1995, Roberts 1996). Tet Q elements integrate into a new host at relatively few specific sites, while the Tet M transposons may integrate in few sites or more randomly into the host chromosome depending on the host. The Tet M transposon can also integrate into plasmids, or within conjugative transposons to create composite elements (Roberts 1996). These composite Gram-positive elements are > 50 kb and have been found in a variety of streptococci and multidrug-resistant *S. pneumoniae* (David et al 1993, Koornhof et al 1992). The prototype of the composite element is Tn*3703*, first described by Clewell et al (1995). Both the composite and the Tet M family of elements can also carry genes which confer resistance to chloramphenicol, erythromycin and kanamycin (Clewell et al 1995).

The *tetM* gene is found in 15 different genera including eight different Gram-negative genera. The *tetO* gene is found in seven Gram-positive and one Gram-negative genera, and *tetS* has been found in two different Gram-positive genera, although it has not been extensively examined in other genera. *tetP* has been found in one genus, but has not been looked for in other genera. We are working on the distribution of *tetQ* and so far have found it in five Gram-positive genera and six Gram-negative species from a variety of ecosystems (Table 3).

The Tet M determinant can transfer between isolates of the same species, between species within the same genus, and between species from very different genera. Examples are given in Table 5. The Tet Q determinant has been shown to transfer between different *Bacteroides* species and related *Provotella* species (Guiney & Hasegawa 1992). More recently we have looked at the host range of the Tet Q determinant: unlike the Tet M determinant it appears to be more common in anaerobic species than facultative or aerobic species (T. Leng & M. C. Roberts, unpublished results). Our preliminary studies are illustrated in Table 3. Whether Tet Q and perhaps Tet S have the potential to become as widespread as Tet M is not clear, but they code for the same mechanism of resistance and are also associated with conjugative elements (Roberts 1996).

Conclusion

The first tetracycline-resistant R-factors were identified 40 years ago in Japan. Since then, tetracycline resistance genes have spread in both Gram-negative and Gram-positive genera, primarily by conjugal transfer of plasmids and/or transposons. The literature has documented the dramatic increase in the number of species and genera which have acquired tetracycline resistance. This has in turn led to a reduction in the efficacy of tetracycline therapy for many diseases. The widespread distribution of specific *tet* genes such as *tetB* or *tetM* (Table 3) supports the hypothesis that the *tet* genes are exchanged by bacteria from many different ecosystems. The presence of

TABLE 4 Distribution of Tet and Otr determinants among *Mycobacterium*, *Nocardia* and *Steptomyces* species

Species	Strain	Tc^{ra}	Tet^b	Otr^c
			Genes	
Mycobacterium avium	ATCC 35712	+	*tetK*	*otrA*
M. avium	ATCC 35718	+	*tetK*	*otrA*
M. avium	MA 1071	ND	*tetK*	ND
M. bovis	ATCC 19120	ND	none	ND
M. intracellulare[d]	MA 531	+	*tetK*	ND
M. intracellulare[d]	MA 577	+	*tetK*	ND
M. intracellulare[d]	MA 968	+	*tetK*	ND
M. intracellulare[d]	MA 1074	+	*tetK*	ND
M. fortuitum	ATCC 6841	–	none	none
M. fortuitum	MF 307	+	none	none
M. fortuitum	MF 414	+	none	none
M. fortuitum third biovariant	ATCC 49403	+	*tetK*	*otrA, otrB*
M. fortuitum third biovariant	ATCC 49404	+	none	none
M. gordonae	MO 16	+	ND	ND
M. beidelbergense[d]	2554/91	ND	*tetL*	ND
M. kansasii	ATCC 12478	+	none	ND
M. kansasii	ATCC 35775	+	none	ND
M. lentiflavum[d]	89-313	ND	*tetK*	ND
M. lentiflavum[d]	89-446	ND	none	ND
M. marinum	ATCC 927	+	none	ND

Organism	Strain	Resistance[a]	tet[b]	otr[c]
M. nonchromogenicum	MO 100	ND	tetK	ND
M. peregrinum	ATCC 14467	+	tetK, tetL	otrA, otrB
M. peregrinum	MP 494	+	none	none
M. scrofulaceum	ATCC 35785	+	none	ND
M. scrofulaceum	ATCC 35793	+	tetK	ND
M. simiae	ATCC 25275	+	none	ND
M. tuberculosis	H37Rv	ND	none	ND
M. tuberculosis	Erdman	ND	none	ND
Mycobacterium spp. [d]	88-885	ND	tetK	ND
Mycobacterium spp. [d]	W58	ND	tetL	ND
Nocardia asteroides	ATCC 19247	+	tetK	ND
N. asteroides	N 394	+	none	ND
N. asteroides	N 410	+	tetK	ND
N. brasiliensis	ATCC 19296	+	none	ND
N. farcinica	N 3318	+	tetK	ND
N. nova	ATCC 33727	+	tetK	ND
N. nova	N 3	+	tetK	ND
N. nova	N 38	+	tetK	ND
Streptomyces spp.	AS 5	+	tetK, tetL	otrA, otrB
Streptomyces spp.	AS 32	+	tetK	otrA, otrB, otrC
Streptomyces spp.	AS 41	+	tetK	otrA, otrB, otrC
Streptomyces spp.	AS 42	+	tetK, tetL	otrA, otrB, otrC
Streptomyces spp.	AS 43	+	tetK, tetL	otrA, otrB
Streptomyces spp.	AS 44	+	tetK	otrA, otrB, otrC
Streptomyces spp.	AS 256	−	none	none

[a]Resistance is designated by + and is defined as a minimum inhibitory concentration (MIC) ≥ 8 mg/ml for tetracycline, and/or doxycyline and/or minocycline; susceptibility is designated by −; ND, the isolate was not tested.

[b]none=not hybridized or no PCR product for tetK, tetL, tetM, tetO or tetS.

[c]none=not hybridized or no PCR product for otrA or otrB and not hybridized with otrC.

[d]Isolates from AIDS patients.

TABLE 5   Mobility of Tet M and Tet Q between different genera

Tet M		Tet Q	
Donor	Recipient	Donor	Recipient
Enterococcus	Bacillus	Bacteroides	Enterococcus
Enterococcus	Butyrivibrio	Prevotella	Enterococcus
Enterococcus	Clostridium		
Enterococcus	Staphylococcus		
Enterococcus	Streptococcus		
Enterococcus	Mycoplasma		
Enterococcus	Acetobacter		
Enterococcus [a]	Alcaligenes		
Enterococcus [a]	Citrobacter		
Enterococcus [a]	Escherichia		
Enterococcus	Pseudomonas		
Streptococcus	Entercoccus		
Listeria	Enterococcus		
Clostridium	Enterococcus		
Fusobacterium	Enterococcus		
Veillonella	Enterococcus		
Bacillus	Clostridium		
Peptostreptococcus	Fusobacterium		
Neisseria [b]	Kingella		
Neisseria [b]	Eikenella		
Neisseria [b]	Haemophilus		
Kingella [b]	Neisseria		
Kingella [b]	Eikenella		
Eikenella [b]	Neisseria		
Escherichia [c]	Bacillus		
Escherichia [c]	Clostridium		
Escherichia [c]	Enterococcus		
Escherichia [c]	Streptococcus		

All transconjugants except where the 25.2 Mda plasmids were present have the *tet*M inserted into the chromosome.
[a] Tn*916* was inserted into the natural plasmid pAD1.
[b] The *tet*M is on an incomplete transposon associated with 25.2 Mda conjugative plasmid which moved rather than the element.
[c] The Tn*916* was on plasmid pAM120 which is a pBR322-derived vector with the cloned intact Tn*916* element.

Gram-positive *tet* genes in natural Gram-negative species supports the hypothesis that Gram-positive genes are being introduced and maintained in Gram-negative species in nature. It is likely that this trend will continue with more Gram-positive genes becoming stably maintained in Gram-negative hosts. Whether the environment can or does influence the ability of bacteria to acquire different *tet* genes is unknown. However, it is likely that an environment where there are large numbers of bacteria with many different species represented provides an excellent climate for gene exchange. Whether or not the *tet* gene is associated with a conjugative element may also influence its distribution. The *tet* genes are found in bacterial pathogens, opportunistic and normal flora species. Significant numbers of normal flora bacteria from a variety of ecosystems are resistant to tetracycline. These may act as reservoirs for antibiotic resistance genes in general and *tet* genes specifically. Over the last 40 years we have seen pathogens become resistant to more and more antibiotics. To help reverse this trend, we will need to reduce the level of antibiotic-resistant bacteria found in the normal flora of humans and animals, in food and the environment.

Acknowledgements

This work was supported in part by National Institutes of Health grants AI24136, DE10913 and USDA/FAS/ICD/RSED Scientific Cooperative Program GM17.

References

Acar JF, Bouanchaud DH, Chabbert YA 1977 Evolutionary aspects of plasmid mediated resistance in a hospital environment. In: Drews J, Hogenauer G Topics in infectious diseases, vol 2: R-factors: their properties and possible control. Springer-Verlag, New York, p 5–23

Andersen SR, Sandaa R-A 1994 Distribution of tetracycline resistance determinants among Gram-negative bacteria isolated from polluted and unpolluted marine sediments. Appl Environ Microbiol 60:908–912

Chopra I, Hawkey PM, Hinton M 1992 Tetracyclines, molecular and clinical aspects. J Antimicrob Chemother 29:245–277

Clewell DB, Flannagan SE, Jaworski DD 1995 Unconstrained bacterial promiscuity: the Tn*916*–Tn*1545* family of conjugative transposons. Trends Microbiol 3:229–236

David F, De Cespedes G, Horaud T 1993 Diversity of chromosomal genetic elements and gene identification in antibiotic resistant strains of *Streptococcus pneumoniae* and *Streptococcus bovis*. Plasmid 29:147–153

Doran JL, Pang Y, Moran AJ et al 1997 *Mycobacterium tuberculosis efpA* encoding a putative efflux protein of the *gacA* drug resistance transporter family. Clin Diag Lab Immun, in press

Falkow S 1975 Infectious multiple drug resistance. Pion, London

Gillespie MT, May JW, Skurray R 1986 Detection of an integrated tetracycline resistance plasmids in the chromosome of methicillin-resistant *Staphylococcus aureus*. J Gen Microbiol 132:1723–1728

Goldstein FW, Kitzis MD Acar JF 1994 N,N-dimethylglycyl-amido derivative of minocycline and 6-dimethyl-6-desoxytetracycline, two new glycylcyclines highly effective against tetracycline-resistant gram-positive cocci. Antimicrob Agents Chemother 38:2218–2220

Guiney DG, Hasegawa P 1992 Transfer of conjugal elements in oral black-pigmented *Bacteroides (Prevotella)* spp. involves DNA rearrangements. J Bacteriol 174:4853–4855

Jones CS, Osborne DJ, Stanley J 1992a Cloning of a probe for a previously undescribed enterobacterial tetracycline resistance gene. Lett Appl Microb 15:106–108

Jones CS, Osborne DJ, Stanley J 1992b Enterobacterial tetracycline resistance in relation to plasmid incompatibility. Mol Cell Probes 6:313–317

Khan SA, Novick RP 1983 Complete nucleotide sequence of pT181, a tetracycline resistance plasmid from *Staphylococcus aureus*. Plasmid 30:163–166

Koornhor HJ, Wasas A, Klugman K 1992 Antimicrobial resistance in *Streptococcus pneumoniae*: a South African perspective. Clin Infect Dis 15:84–94

Levy SB 1992 The antibiotic paradox: how miracle drugs are destroying the miracle. Plenum, New York

Li L-Y, Shoemaker NB, Salyers AA 1995 Location and characteristics of the transfer region of *Bacteriodes* conjugative transposon and regulation of transfer genes. J Bacteriol 177:4992–4999

Mendez B, Tachibana C, Levy SB 1980 Heterogeneity of tetracycline resistance determinants. Plasmid 3:99–108

Needham C, Rahman M, Dyke KGH, Noble WC 1994 An investigation of plasmids from *Staphylococcus aureus* that mediate resistance to mupirocin and tetracycline. Microbiol 140:2577–2583

Pang Y, Bosch T, Roberts MC 1994a Single polymerase chain reaction for the detection of tetracycline resistant determinants Tet K and Tet L. Mol Cell Probes 8:417–422

Pang Y, Brown BA, Steingrube VA, Wallace RJ Jr, Roberts MC 1994b Tetracycline resistance determinants in *Mycobacterium* and *Streptomyces* species. Antimicrob Agents Chemother 38:1408–1412

Projan SJ, Novick R 1988 Comparative analysis of five related staphylococcal plasmids. Plasmid 19:203–221

Roberts MC 1989a Gene transfer in the urogenital and respiratory tract. In: Levy S, Miller RV (eds) Gene transfer in the environment. McGraw-Hill, New York, p 347–375

Roberts MC 1989b Plasmid-mediated Tet M in *Haemophilus ducreyi*. Antimicrob Agents Chemother 33:1611–1613

Roberts MC 1994 Epidemiology of tetracycline resistance determinants. Trends Microbiol 2:353–357

Roberts MC 1996 Tetracycline-resistant determinants: mechanisms of action, regulation of expression, genetic mobility, and distribution. FEMS Microbiol Rev 19:1–24

Roberts MC, Pang Y, Spencer RC, Winstanley TG, Brown BA, Wallace RJ Jr 1991 Tetracycline resistance in *Moraxella (Branhamella)* catarrhalis — demonstration of two clonal outbreaks using pulsed-field gel electrophoresis. Antimicrob Agents Chemother 35:2453–2455

Roberts MC, Chung W, Roe DE 1996 Characterization of tetracycline and erythromycin determinants in *Treponema denticola*. Antimicrob Agents Chemother 40:1690–1694

Roe DE, Roberts MC, Braham P, Weinberg A 1995 Characterization of tetracycline resistance in *Actinobacillus actinomycetemcomitans*. Oral Microbiol Immunol 10:227–232

Sakaguchi R, Shishido K 1988 Molecular cloning of a tetracycline-resistance determinant from *Bacillus subtilis* chromosomal DNA and its expression in *Escherichia coli* and *B. subtilis*. Biochim Biophys Acta 949:9–57

Watanabe T 1963 Infectious heredity of multiple drug resistance in bacteria. Bacteriol Rev 27:87–115

Wasteson Y, Roe DE, Falk K, Roberts MC 1996 Characterization of antibiotic resistance in *Actinobacillus pleuropneumoniae*. Vet Microbiol 48:41–50

DISCUSSION

Davies: I have read recently that *Nocardia* (an **act**inomycete) is an emerging pathogen. It has been shown to cause infection by replication or survival in macrophages and there are predictions that it is going to be a difficult bug in the future. It is interesting that *Nocardia* strains already carry tetracycline resistance.

Baquero: It is not a pathogen to worry too much about. We see it about once a year, and mainly in immunosuppressed patients.

Cohen: Several years ago we had an outbreak of *Nocardia* in persons who went to an island to get injections of some animal materials that were supposed to help their immunosuppressive diseases and/or keep them young. They got systemic *Nocardia* infections.

Lerner: The use of intensive immunocompromising therapy is going to be expanding, particularly now that insurance will pay for it: for instance, bone marrow transplantation for breast cancer, a very common disease, is going to be utilized more frequently.

Bennish: Hospitals are steadily becoming one big ICU. The intensity of antimicrobial therapy given the degree of immunosuppression is logs ahead of what it was when I did my training.

Summers: Why is it that *tet* loci don't tend to occur in the integron? They are just single genes aren't they?

Hall: It is possibly because *tet* loci have already found a successful mechanism for inter-genome transfer and have already spread round quite effectively. However, I would be reluctant to suggest that the *tet* gene couldn't get into a cassette.

Roberts: The *tet* loci are also found on transposons, so they aren't immobile.

Levy: It is of interest that the membrane efflux determinant in an integron is *cmlA* — which has its own promoter that presumably controls its expression. Too much production of such a membrane protein can be lethal to bacteria. These kinds of potentially toxic mechanisms are not going to be wanted in a system that is controlling so many different other resistances.

Hall: I assume you are referring to the toxic effects of efflux proteins. In the case of *cmlA* it has a promoter, but it also has a translation attenuation system to keep it switched off. So, it is only expressed in response to chloramphenicol exposure.

Skurray: I should remind you that *qacE*, which is associated with integrons and gives partial resistance to antiseptics and disinfectants, does encode an efflux system (Paulsen et al 1993).

Hall: The complete *qacE* gene that is in a cassette, in Tn*402*, is an efflux protein. This cassette also contains a weak promoter, and we need to look at whether its expression is regulated.

Skurray: I'm intrigued by the number of *tetK* genes that are being isolated in Gram-positive and Gram-negative bacteria. Are the determinants you have commented on highly homologous in sequence with the classical Tet K from staphylococci?

Roberts: The problem is that not a lot of sequencing has been done for other *tetK* genes. We have just a few available in GenBank and they are highly related.

Skurray: How are they encoded?

Roberts: Most of these look like they're not associated in plasmids. We don't see plasmids. However, one complication is that it is hard to detect them in these organisms (mycobacteria) even if you know that they have them. Tentatively, therefore, I would say that they appear to be chromosomal.

Skurray: It is interesting that some cells carry multiple tetracycline resistance determinants; for example, staphylococcal strains may have two or three different tetracycline resistance determinants. Maybe there is some feature about tetracycline resistance that provides an additional advantage to the cell over the resistance itself.

Roberts: The Gram-positives tend to carry multiple Tet determinants, and they may be of the same type, such as two effluxes, or they may have efflux and ribosomal protection. Thus, you might have an isolate carrying a *tetK* and *tetL* genes or *tetK* and *tetM* genes.

Skurray: The idea of a bacterial cell having multiple efflux systems seems to be particularly important; some bacteria, such as *E. coli*, naturally carry on their chromosomes a number of multidrug resistance export genes with a wide variety of substrate specificities. One has to ask what the significance of such an apparent redundancy is. Possibly these efflux systems provide the cell with resistance to naturally encountered toxins, say in the host cell (for a recent review see Paulsen et al 1996).

Levy: In several studies in which antibiotics have been removed, tetracycline resistance may be the last to go. We have always assumed that this is because it is regulated and so does not have a large cost to the host. In fact, Richard Lenski's results suggest that the Tet determinant is so important during chloramphenicol selection that a strong relationship has been formed with its host.

Lenski: Yes, and if you do get rid of the tetracycline resistance, then the cell is unhappy. It is clearly doing something beneficial for the cell. We came up with two classes of explanation for how such an efflux mechanism could benefit the cell even in the absence of antibiotic. The first is that the efflux mechanism has been usurped and is being used by the cell to rid itself of some toxic metabolite, for example. The other is that bacteria are constantly evolving, and it may be that having these efflux proteins stuck into the cell membrane is vital in terms of modifying the expression or configuration of other membrane proteins. Thus, the efflux mechanism has become part of the milieu in which all the other membrane-associated functions have to operate. So, if the efflux proteins are suddenly removed, these other functions are also disrupted.

Levy: Tet resistance determinants, which have very low K_m for tetracycline, may do other things. For instance, some help in K^+ transport (Dosch et al 1984) and some, at high pH, help in Na^+/H^+ exchange (Guffanti & Krulwich 1995).

Baquero: Is antibiotic resistance generally selecting the elements involved in gene mobility? In other words, is the absolute number of elements involved in gene mobility increasing because of antibiotics? This would accelerate the rate of evolution.

Lenski: Yes. It seems to me that the two processes are linked. When you select for antibiotic resistance, an additional mobile element is introduced into the genetic background, which creates more opportunity for further spread of both the resistance gene and the mobile element. It creates a sort of autocatalytic process.

Summers: Tn*10*-type Tet resistance is also associated with some alteration in metal ion transport (Bochner et al 1980). Taking Richard's point about the adaptation as an 'ensemble' phenomenon, once you've got addicted to this particular thing you can't let go because you've adapted some other important system to require it.

Levy: There are two open reading frames (ORFs) on Tn*10* that we found highly conserved in all Tn*10*-like elements which are associated with tetracycline resistance (P. Flynn, S. Anderson, K. Schollmeier, W. Hillen & S. B. Levy, unpublished data). One of these ORFs (the so-called ORF-R) strongly resembles the transcriptional activator MarA, which elicits multidrug resistance. When others have deleted part of the transposon they saw no change in tetracycline resistance. However, when we have overproduced the product we have seen low level Mar-like resistance. Thus, besides tetracycline resistance, Tn*10* might be doing something more.

Hall: Are you saying that the *tet* transcriptional activator may be cross-talking in the same way that *marA* and *soxS* do?

Levy: It may be doing something else to the cell independent of the tetracycline resistance, because it's so highly conserved.

Davies: It is worth mentioning that the study of tetracycline resistance has led to some positive benefits. The tetracycline repressor combined with tetracycline is probably one of the most effective means of regulating gene expression in eukaryotes.

Levy: It scares me, however, that it is also being used in plant systems as the means of turning on genes. What concerns me in particular is whether it will ever be considered as a means to keep plants better by producing tetracycline.

Cohen: In many plants another antibiotic, kanamycin, is used for selecting recombinant strains: the potential for abuse here is that in order to assist survival of the recombinants, one could use kanamycin in the field.

Davies: On the other hand, without studies of R plasmids there would never have been any biotechnology as we know it today.

Piddock: There are fewer Tet elements in Gram-negative than Gram-positive bacteria. Perhaps this is because of the *marRAB* locus in Gram-negative bacteria which mediates tetracycline resistance, and thus there may not be the selective pressure for multiple determinants.

Roberts: You can have chromosomal β-lactamases and plasmid-encoded genes which are different. Thus a single cell can still carry multiple genes.

Piddock: But one often sees the lack of outer membrane proteins which may indicate the involvement of *marRAB*. This has not been examined in any depth.

Summers: Is there a homologue of *mar* in Gram-positives?

Levy: We don't know.

Levin: Some years ago, George Armelagos and his collaborators presented evidence for tetracycline in the bones of ancient Nubians (Bassett et al 1980). Presumably they obtained this tetracycline by eating streptomycin-contaminated stored foods. One implication of this is that long before we began to use antibiotics for clinical purposes, there was already selection for antibiotic-resistant human pathogenic and commensal bacteria.

References

Bassett EJ, Keith MS, Armelagos GJ, Martin DL, Villanueva AR 1980 Tetracycline-labeled human bone from ancient Sudanese Nubia (A.D. 350). Science 209:1532–1534

Bochner BR, Huang H-C, Schieven GL, Ames BN 1980 Positive selection for loss of tetracycline resistance. J Bacteriol 143:926–933

Dosch DC, Salvacion FF, Epstein W 1984 Tetracycline resistance element of pBR322 mediates potassium transport. J Bacteriol 160:1188–1190

Guffanti AA, Krulwich TA 1995 Tetracycline/H^+ antiport and Na^+/H^+ antiport catalysed by the *Bacillus subtilis* TetA(L) transporter expressed in *Escherichia coli*. J Bacteriol 177:4557–4561

Paulsen IT, Littlejohn TG, Radstrom P et al 1993 The 3' conserved segment of integrons contains a gene associated with multidrug resistance to antiseptics and disinfectants. Antimicrob Agents Chemother 37:761–768

Paulsen IT et al 1996 Proton-dependent multidrug efflux systems. Microbiol Rev 60, in press

DATE DUE